# *Lavender Oil*

# Lavender Oil

## THE NEW GUIDE TO NATURE'S MOST
## VERSATILE TRADITIONAL REMEDY

### Julia Lawless

**Thorsons**
*An Imprint of HarperCollinsPublishers*

*Dedicated to Natasha*

Thorsons
An Imprint of HarperCollins*Publishers*
77–85 Fulham Palace Road,
Hammersmith, London W6 8JB
1160 Battery Street,
San Francisco, California 94111–1213

Published by Thorsons 1994
5 7 9 10 8 6 4

© Julia Lawless 1994

Julia Lawless asserts the moral right to
be identified as the author of this work

A catalogue record for this book
is available from the British Library

ISBN 0 7225 3031 5

Printed and bound in Great Britain by
Caledonian International Book Manufacturing Ltd, Glasgow

# Contents

Acknowledgements      vii

Lavender Oil – An Introduction      ix

*PART I: Lavender's Medical and
Historical Background*      1

1 The Scent of Times Past      3
2 A Traditional European Folk Remedy      10
3 Modern Medical Evidence      16
4 Production, Chemical Composition
  and Quality Control      26
5 Summary of the Properties and
  Applications of Lavender Oil      33
6 Methods of Use, Safety Data and
  Storage Precautions      39

**PART II: A-Z of Health Care Applications**     45

Abscesses & boils (furuncle); acne & spots; anxiety; arthritis & gout; asthma; bruises & bumps; burns; carbuncles; chickenpox; children's ailments; cracked skin; cuts & wounds; cystitis & urethritis; depression; dermatitis & eczema; disinfectant uses; dyspepsia (indigestion) & flatulence; earache; epilepsy; fatigue; hair care; headaches; herpes; high blood-pressure (hypertension); immune system; impetigo; infectious illness; insect bites & stings; insomnia; jetlag; laryngitis; leucorrhoea & pruritis; lice (pediculosis); menopause; migraine; mood swings & hysteria; muscular aches & pains; nausea; palpitations (tachycardia); period pains; perfume uses; perspiration; pregnancy & childbirth; pre-menstrual tension; rheumatism; scabies; shock & vertigo; skin care; splinters; sprains; stress; sunburn; ulcers; whooping cough.

Appendix A: The different Types of
Lavender Oil     111

Appendix B: The Constituents of
Lavender Oil     115

References     118
Bibliography     121
Useful Addresses     124
Index     126

# Acknowledgements

As I write, the lavender in my garden is just coming into full bloom. It is one of my favourite herbs: sturdy yet delicate, with a mass of hazy-purple flowers which suffuse the air with their dreamy-soft fragrance. I am also very fond of the essential oil of lavender, and use it more than any other oil about the house. It is ideal as a remedy for children, for the treatment of all sorts of minor ailments, and as a bath oil or room fragrance. This book is dedicated to my young daughter Natasha, who has a keen interest in all perfumes and loves the scent of lavender.

I would especially like to thank the following people, who have contributed in various ways to the completion of this book:

Steward Alcock for his excellent translations from the French; John Black for his expertise and for providing technical information; Cara Denman for her guidance; Jane Graham-Maw and those at

Thorsons for their sympathetic approach to the project; Len Smith for his editorial comments; and my husband Alec for his ongoing support.

I would also like to thank *Perfumer & Flavorist* for their kind permission to reprint the table outlining the detailed constituents of lavender oil (see Appendix B).

# *Lavender Oil —*
# *An Introduction*

*Oh how happy I am not to be one of those ornamental flowers that decorate the border! I'm not at risk of falling into uncouth hands and am sheltered from frivolous discourse.*

*Unlike my sisters, the plants, nature makes me grow far from streams, and I don't like cultivated gardens or land.*

*I am wild. Far from society, my sojourn is spent in deserts and solitude, for I don't like mixing with the crowd!*

*...Free, I am free!*

'THE SONG OF LAVENDER' (*'La Chante de la Lavande'*)'

The unique character or personality of lavender is evident from the words of this song, taken from *A Thousand and One Nights*. Originally a native of the Mediterranean region, growing at altitudes of up to 1,800 metres (nearly 6,000 feet) in the mountains of southern France, this beautiful yet

tough and resilient plant has been cherished by all
cultures alike, not only for its fine fragrance but
also its valuable medicinal properties. It is one of
the few herbs that has never gone out of fashion,
for it has enjoyed widespread use from the earliest
times to the present day. Lavender has always been
a favourite!

Lavenders make up a small group or genus
(*lavendula*) containing about 30 different species
within the botanical family *Labiatae*. Several
varieties of lavender are used medicinally, but the
most valuable is the common or 'true' lavender
*L. angustifolia*, also known as *L. officinalis* and *L.
vera*. This hardy, evergreen shrub which grows to
a height of about 1 m (3½ ft) becomes increasingly
woody and spreading with age, and has a sweeter,
more refined fragrance than any of the other
varieties. Today, 'true' lavender can be found
growing wild in Italy (Calabria), France (especially
in Provence), on the eastern coast of Spain and
right into North Africa. It is also commonly found
in cultivated form throughout the rest of Europe
as well as in India, Australia and the US.

It is generally assumed that the Romans were
the first to introduce lavender to Britain, although
the exact date of its arrival remains uncertain. *The
Feate of Gardening* written by Jon Gardener in
about 1440 mentions a plant called 'lavyndull'
already growing in English gardens at the turn of

take a scientific approach to phytotherapy (herbal medicine) and aromatherapy.

In England, on the other hand, essential oils and herbal remedies are still viewed mainly with suspicion by most pharmacists and general practitioners, or dismissed as something 'quirky' or 'old-fashioned', in spite of growing popular interest. Aromatherapy in England has consequently developed along different lines from that of the French model, and is seen more as a 'complementary' type of therapy than a 'main-stream' clinical treatment. In Britain, aromatherapy is mainly the province of qualified aromatherapists, most of whom also use massage as a central part of their work, making it particularly suited to stress-related problems or psychosomatic conditions.

Aromatherapy could therefore be said to have developed into three interrelated forms or practices:

1. Clinical Aromatherapy – principally practised in France
2. Aromatherapy Massage – principally practised in the UK
3. Home Aromatherapy – in the tradition of 'herbal simples', i.e. easy-to-use houschold remedies that can be used to treat a variety of common ailments.

This book touches on all three areas, especially the last, for lavender oil has been used as a household remedy for centuries and its various applications have been tried and tested over time. It is a very safe oil which can be used easily for first-aid purposes as well as for a wide variety of common problems such as skin complaints, respiratory disorders, muscular pains and children's illnesses. Its classic floral fragrance lifts the spirits; its soothing anti-depressant properties are ideally suited to the stressful climate of late-20th-century life.

The type of lavender oil that is most commonly available, and the type which is referred to here, comes from the 'true' lavender (*L. angustifolia*, *L. officinalis*, *L. vera*), also known as 'Old English Lavender'. There are, however, many varieties of lavender, each having its own characteristics: for example, the oil of aspic or spike lavender (*L. latifolia*) and lavandin (*L.* x *intermedia*) have a more stimulating effect than that of 'true' lavender. A comparison of these different types of lavender can be found in Appendix A at the end of this book.

# PART I

# Lavender's Medical and Historical Background

# The Scent of Times Past

Lavender has been a popular perfume material since ancient times. In ancient Egypt and Turkey lavender was valued for its clean, refreshing scent, while Arab women once used the oil to add lustre to their hair. The Romans used lavender to scent their bath water, and its name is generally thought to have derived from the Latin *lavare* – to wash. The early Greeks also thought highly of its fragrance; Dioscorides is reported to have said that:

> *Oil of lavender, when made by passing flowers through a glass alembic [i.e. when distilled], surpasses all other perfumes.*

According to Greek myth, lavender was also one of the herbs dedicated to Hecate, the Goddess of witches and enchantment. Conversely, throughout Europe a sprig of lavender was believed to avert 'the evil eye' and it was commonly strewn in churches and dwelling places, especially on the feast days of St Barnabas and St Paul.

Lavender remained in great demand throughout this ancient period, both in its fresh and dried form. From medieval times in Europe, the dried flowers were used in pot-pourris, 'tussie mussies', sweet-bags and for laying among clothes and linen to keep moths away. In Tudor times it was also used to stuff quilted jackets and caps – during the reign of Queen Elizabeth I it was common for women to sew little sachets of lavender into their skirts. Sprigs of fresh lavender or woodruff were bound into bundles and laid upon pillows or hung in homes as air fresheners in both Elizabethan England and the American colonies.

Essential oils (or 'chymical oils' as they were called) were beginning to make an appearance at this time, but prior to the 16th century there are few records of the process of distillation taking place using native herbs. One remarkable exception to this rule can be found in the *Meddygon Myddfai*, a famous little collection of remedies and charms written by the celebrated Welsh physicians of Myddfai in Carmarthen round about the middle of the 13th century. In it there is a recipe for 'aqua water', concocted from lavender, rosemary, thyme, fennel and parsley roots ground together in a mortar, sprinkled with a little salt and then placed in a still with some red or white wine. This was then placed in a pot full of ashes on a slow burning furnace...

*and so do stylle hyt al to-gedre; then take thye water*
*that is distillyd, and distyllet azen zyf you wolte and*
*use that of euerech day a lytel sponeful fastyng.*

It was only after the publication of the *Grete Herball*
in 1526, however, a book which included
illustrations of the retorts and stills used for the
extraction of essential oils, that the English began
to experiment extensively with their own native
flora. By the late 16th century, following the
Continental lead, it had become fashionable to
have one's own 'stillroom'. The production of
various aromatic preparations soon became part of
the routine in all large houses. Stillroom secrets
were sometimes recorded in special books along
with personal recipes, or were passed down orally
from generation to generation. A great deal of
time and expertise went into this work, which was
usually carried out by the mistress of the house
together with other women...

*from fields they gathered rushes and sweet-smelling*
*grasses to throw on their floors; in the garden they*
*cultivated medicinal and aromatic herbs; and in their*
*still rooms, they powdered, mixed and stilled,*
*transforming the summer's harvest into moth bags,*
*sweet-waters, pot-pourris, sweet-bags, pomanders, wash-*
*balls, sachets, herb-pillows, tussie-mussies, vinegars and*
*teas.*[1]

The earliest known recipe for a composite

lavender water, dated 1615, gives directions for distilling the flowers together with canella, wallflower, gallingall and grains of paradise. These early forms of extraction were carried out by the process of water distillation – the flowers being literally immersed in a container of water which was then heated so the aromatic oils were carried over in a condenser with the water vapour. The distillate then separated out into two layers, with the volatile oil on top. Increasingly during the 17th century, as the knowledge of distillation spread throughout Britain, a variety of different essential oils were produced. These were blended to form exquisite natural perfumes and various 'sweet waters', which were commonly presented as gifts. Lavender water remained one of the most popular English scents

> *There are certain types of women whose individuality seems to be better expressed by the use of lavender water than by any other scent. Gracious gentlewomen, with a love of all that is fair, harmonious and beautiful in life and thought, rather than the sophisticated, dashing type...* [2]

Queen Victoria herself had a particular fondness for the smell of lavender, and the royal apartments were redolent with its sweet, refreshing scent. Her Majesty is said to have purchased the essential oil direct from a lady who distilled it herself for use throughout the household as a domestic disinfectant. Furniture was also rubbed with lavender oil, as a forerunner of modern wax and polish. It was also used to scent gloves, leather goods and women's hair. Indeed, the Victorian age as a whole demonstrated a penchant for lavender, and it was frequently mentioned in honeyed Victorian verse. An Elizabethan love song called 'Lavender's Blue' re-emerged over 100 years later as the popular Victorian nursery rhyme:

> *Lavender's blue, dilly, dilly, lavender's green;*
> *When I am king, dilly, dilly, you shall be queen...*

For many, the scent of lavender still has a nostalgic quality...it is 'the fragrance of half-forgotten things'³ . It tends to suggest a naïve, innocent quality, bringing back recollections of balmy summer days spent outdoors as a child, the comforting aroma of freshly laundered sheets, or the lingering trace of lavender water on a woman's sleeve, even though her features may have long since faded with time:

> *And still she slept an azure-lidded sleep,*
> *In blanched linen, smooth, and lavender'd*

> > 'EVE OF SAINT AGNES'
> > JOHN KEATS (1819)

Lavender is often considered an old-fashioned perfume, associated with grandmothers and great-aunts — indeed, a heart-shaped lavender sachet made from pink net and tied with a velvet ribbon was once a traditional gift from a maiden aunt to her young nieces. But the 'old maid' image is not entirely fair — after all, it was once worn extensively by prostitutes to advertise their trade and attract customers! Yet through its rich associations lavender continues to have a strong traditional appeal, and it remains in huge demand by the perfumery industry today.

> *According to Priest, good lavender oil is one of the most enjoyable raw materials that a perfumer has to work with. At once powerful and delicate...it is seldom used alone but serves in many blends imparting a delightfully fresh and sweet note. It blends excellently with the citrus oils, especially bergamot, to produce colognes of all types...*[4]

Yardley, one of the oldest perfume companies in the world, was founded on products based principally on lavender! They produced their first lavender soap during the reign of Charles I, and after the First World War they became the world's largest manufacturer of lavender products. Since 1936 Norfolk Lavender Ltd, England's largest and oldest lavender farm, has supplied Yardley with lavender oil for the manufacture of lavender water, lavender soap and other products, including their classic scent 'Lavender' (first produced in

1913). Other examples of quality perfumes which contain old English lavender are 'Blue Grass', 'Paco Rabanne' and 'Silvestre', as well as many fougere-type fragrances.

# A Traditional
# European Folk Remedy

Lavender has been used for healing purposes since primitive times, but the first mention of its specific use can be traced back to ancient Greece. Dioscorides is credited with having compiled the first extensive *Materia Medica* during the 1st century AD, in which he described the therapeutic qualities of over 500 plants taken from both Egyptian and Greek herbal lore. He refers to French lavender (*L. stoechas*) as:

> *An herb with slender twiggs having ye haire like Tyme, but yet longer leaved...sharp in ye taste and somewhat bitterish, but ye decoction of it as the Hyssop is good for ye griefs in ye thorax...*[1]

Dioscorides also attributed certain laxative and invigorating properties to it, and recommended its use in a tea-like infusion for chest complaints. The great doctor Galen (AD 129–199) prescribed French lavender as an antidote to poisons, and for uterine disorders. Pliny the Elder, a contemporary of Dioscorides, used it for promoting menstruation and for treating snake bites and stings as well as, when taken in wine, for digestive, liver, renal and gall bladder disorders. He also ascribed it with some psychological benefit by claiming that it banished the 'pain of the bereft'. Indeed,

> ...*from the Greek medical practice there is derived the term 'iatralypte', from the physician who cured by the use of aromatic unctions.*[2]

But whereas the Greeks regarded lavender principally as a medicine, the Romans used it extensively for its fragrance. Pliny was the first to distinguish between French lavender (*L. stoechas*) and 'true' lavender (*L. vera*), revealing that the Romans used the latter for 'stretching' exotic perfumes. The Romans spent vast sums of money on their ritual ablutions, and at the public baths the *Unctuarium* or 'Oil Room' housed innumerable ready-mixed lotions, many of which contained lavender. The Romans also traditionally used the dried crushed leaves of lavender as a form of incense in honour of their gods. It was burnt on hot coals at ceremonial occasions as well as in preparation for childbirth.

It was the monks who preserved the knowledge of herbal lore in Europe during the Dark Ages. The Abbess of Hildegarde (1098–1180) from the diocese of Mainz made some of the earliest

medicinal references to lavender in her prolific
writings. She dedicated a whole chapter to
lavender, which she described as a fierce, dry and
strong-smelling herb, albeit without edible value.[3]
She prescribed it for, among other things, clearing
the eyes, getting rid of lice and banishing evil
spirits! She also recommended lavender for
'keeping a pure character'.

The monasteries, in addition, cultivated
elaborately laid out herb gardens behind their high
walls. A special plot was usually designated for the
herb garden near the kitchen, which was often
planted with a single herb in each bed, grown
especially for its specific culinary or medicinal use.
This type of classically arranged formal herb
garden lasted right up to the mid-17th century,
and reached a peak of popularity during the
Elizabethan era. In *A Winter's Tale*, Shakespeare
describes a few of the herbs one might expect to
find growing in such a garden:

> *Hot lavender, mints, savory, marjoram;*
> *The marigold, that goes to bed wi' the sun,*
> *And with him rises weeping; these are flowers*
> *Of middle summer...*

Throughout this period, lavender was employed
principally as a domestic household item and as a
medicinal agent. It was also occasionally used for
culinary purposes, especially as a flavouring for

vinegar. The dried powder was sometimes added to dishes as a condiment to 'comfort the stomach', and Queen Elizabeth I apparently enjoyed a conserve of lavender.

William Turner, often called the Father of English Botany, wrote a pioneering work on herbalism between 1538 and 1568 which he dedicated to Elizabeth I. In this *New Herball* he recommended true lavender for all diseases of the brain that 'come of a cold cause', and lavender water for 'dulness of the head'.

All the early European herbalists were in general agreement that true lavender was particularly effective for nervous complaints, and that its fragrance alone could combat melancholy and comfort and revive the spirits. John Gerard, writing at the end of the 16th century, claimed that:

> The distilled water of lavender smelt unto, or the temples and forehead bathed therewith, is a refreshing to them that have the Catalepsy, a light migram, and to them that have the falling sicknesse, and that use to swoune much...[1]

while 50 years later, John Parkinson confirmed that lavender was 'especiall good use for all griefes and paines of the head and brain'. In *Culpeper's Complete Herbal*, the well-known astrologically based treatise first published in 1652, the author describes lavender in the following terms:

> *Mercury owns this herb. It is of especial use in pains of the head and brain which proceed from cold, apoplexy, falling-sickness, the dropsy, or sluggish malady, cramps, convulsions, palsies and often faintings...the tremblings and passions of the heart, and faintings and swoonings, applied to the temples or nostrils, to be smelt unto...*[5]

Culpeper also recommended lavender for digestive upsets or weakness, liver and spleen obstructions, menstrual problems, toothache or the loss of voice, but he warned that Oil of Spike should be used with care due to its 'hot and subtle spirit'.

Reports on the virtues of lavender reached a peak with William Salmon's herbal of 1710, in which he described 12 different preparations using lavender for various diseases of the head, brain, nerves and womb. Its many properties were listed by Salmon as:

> *Abstersive, Aperitive, Astringent, Discursive, Dieuretic, and Incisive...Cephalick, Neurotick, Stomatick, Cordial, Nephretick and Hysterick. It is Alexipharmic, Analeptick and Antiparatitick, being of very subtle and thin parts.*[6]

The 18th century saw interest in traditional folk remedies begin to wane, however, in the growing light of chemical science. Over the next two centuries the use of lavender as a remedy dwindled, as people put their faith in the newly developed medicines and drugs. It was only in the mid-20th century that herbal remedies began to be re-assessed seriously in modern scientific terms.

# Modern Medical Evidence

In 1931, with the publication of *A Modern Herbal*
Mrs M. Grieve drew modern scientific knowledge
and traditional folklore together for the first time
into a comprehensive encyclopaedia. In this
pioneering work she describes over a thousand
British and American plants, providing information
on their exact botanical origin, cultivation,
chemical and medicinal properties as well as their
historical usage. Like the early herbalists, Mrs
Grieve viewed lavender principally as a nervine,
and she recommended the oil, rubbed on the
temples, for mental depression, delusions and
nervous headaches. However, she also drew attention to its powerful antiseptic and germicidal
properties, for which it was gaining increasing
recognition, especially in France:

> *Its use in the swabbing of wounds obtained further
> proof during the War, and the French Academy of*

> Medicine is giving attention to the oil for this and
> other antiseptic surgical purposes. The oil is successfully
> used in the treatment of sores, varicose ulcers, burns
> and scalds. In France it is a regular thing for most
> households to keep a bottle of Essence of Lavender as a
> domestic remedy against bruises, bites and trivial aches
> and pains, both external and internal.[1]

Indeed, the French have long been familiar with
the benefits of lavender, and it is to France that
one must look for the first scientific reports on the
clinical use of lavender oil. During the First World
War, applications of aromatic essences were
common in a variety of civilian and military
hospitals. In 1915 the French physician Mencière
was treating war wounds using various compositions of essential oils, including lavender, due
to their remarkable bactericidal and healing
properties.

Dr Jean Valnet, another wartime surgeon,
commented on the antiseptic and cicatrizing
(wound-healing) properties of essential oils,
especially those found among the *Labiatae* family
such as lavender, sage, thyme and rosemary. He
noted that the antiseptic power of lavender was
stronger than that of phenol, cresol or guiaicol,
and that its vapour destroyed pneumococcus and
haemolytic streptococcus in 12–24 hours. He also
found that lavender essence killed the tuberculosis
bacillus at a strength of 0.2 per cent, the Eberth's

bacillus (typhoid) and staphylococcus at 4.5 per cent, and Loeffler's bacillus (diphtheria) at 5 per cent.[2] Valnet recommended the administering of vaporized lavender oil in a 2 per cent solution for disinfecting sick rooms, clinics and operating theatres; he also expounded upon the anti-toxic, pesticidal, antispasmodic, sedative and emmen-agogic properties of lavender.

But it was the French perfumer, René-Maurice Gattefossé (1881–1950) who did the most to draw attention to the potential of lavender oil during this period. Through his research work, Gattefossé had become increasingly fascinated by the numerous essential oil preparations used by the peasants and natives as folk remedies. The value of their traditional knowledge was validated when Gattefossé suffered serious burns to his hands in a laboratory explosion and found that simply by applying dressings of pure lavender oil, he was able successfully to heal the wound in a short period of time, and prevent scarring. After this encouraging result he devoted much of his time to exploring and promoting the therapeutic use of aromatics. In 1932 he published a paper in the journal *Parfum Modern* specifically on the antiseptic role of lavender, and in 1937 he published his two main works, *Aromathérapie* and *Antiseptiques Essentiales*. These books had a profound impact on the scientific establishment regarding the medical use of essential oils in general, and it is from Gattefossé that the modern term 'Aromatherapy' originated.

In *Aromathérapie*, Gattefossé cites numerous case histories involving a variety of conditions including battle injuries, burns, varicose ulcers, venereal sores, gangrene and atonic wounds which were treated almost exclusively with pure lavender oil (or in a solution), with excellent results. He concludes:

> In all cases the following is noted: rapid disappearance of pus; decrease in the number of bacteria; powerful stimulation of healing; recovery in a very short time. It is as though the physiological matter receives an added dynamism causing the pathological phenomena to abate immediately.[3]

The work of Gattefossé was taken up by Marguerite Maury (1895–1968) in France after the Second World War. Mme Maury was a dedicated and inspired woman who did much to establish the reputation of aromatherapy. She set up the first aromatherapy clinics in Paris, Britain and Switzerland and was awarded two international prizes (in 1962 and 1967 respectively) for her studies on essential oils and cosmetology. In her research work she focused on the rejuvenating properties of essential oils, the results of which were published in English as *The Secret of Life and*

*Youth* (1964). From her writing it is clear that she valued lavender primarily as a skin care agent and a 'restorer of balance', but also as a nerve tonic:

> *In cases of great exhaustion, of fatigue caused by physical effort, or excessive barometric changes, a friction with pure lavender essences without spirits works wonders.*[4]

Mme Maury also emphasized the psychological impact of fragrance and the importance of choosing the correct oils for each patient so as to make a personalized blend or 'individual prescription'. Her work in many ways set the tone for aromatherapy as it developed in the UK, not only as a beauty therapy with its emphasis on skin care, but also as a treatment for stress and nervous/emotional disorders.

For in Britain, unlike France, aromatic oils are used principally by 'complementary' practitioners – notably by aromatherapists – and increasingly by nurses working in hospital wards. This helps to explain why the majority of 'field' studies carried out in the UK have been undertaken by independent researchers or by nurses, rather than by medical doctors as in France. Such studies have tended to concentrate on the nervine, analgesic and sedative properties of lavender oil, applied externally through massage, baths or simply by inhalation.

Lavender is an oil which has undergone a considerable amount of research in the past few years, and is in fact the most frequently used essential oil in hospitals in the UK today:

## * 1988

– In one Oxford hospital, lavender oil has been used for a number of years to help patients sleep at night, either by giving them a lavender bath or by sprinkling a little oil on their bedclothes. Lavender has also been used to enhance analgesia (pain-relief) in cases of arthritis, muscular tension and muscle spasm. One patient who had an amputation below the knee enjoyed almost complete relief from pain for 90 minutes after being massaged on his upper leg with diluted lavender oil. In addition, the scent of lavender was found to help patients relax before surgery and prolong the effect of any pre-operative medication.

*Here is clinical evidence that essential oils can potentiate the effects of sedative drugs, so by using both together the same effect can be achieved with a lower dose.*[5]

## * 1989

– The neurodepressive effects of lavender oil have been backed up by experimental research tests in the laboratory. In one study, lavender oil was diluted to

1 part in 60 with olive oil and then given orally to mice. The mice were then required to perform a number of tests; sedative effects were observed. It was also found that a significant interaction existed with pentabarbital, in that sleeping time was increased and wakefulness reduced.[6]

> Lavender oil has also exhibited CNS-depressive activities on experimental animals (e.g. mice). Such activities include anticonvulsive effects, inhibition of the spontaneous motor activity, and the initiation of the narcotic effects of chloral hydrate.[7]

## * 1991
— In another study carried out at the Old Manor Hospital in Salisbury, England, Mark Hardy RMN conducted an experiment to assess the effects of lavender oil on the sleeping patterns of elderly mentally ill patients, in place of their usual medication. In these initial tests he used a vortex air freshener to vaporize the lavender oil into the wards at night, with excellent results:

> Residents exhibited less restlessness during the night, their sleep was deeper and so they were not being awakened while staff made their rounds, there were fewer periods of simple insomnia and the mood of residents on waking was more pleasant...There was even a slight increase in the hours of sleep obtained using lavender oil as opposed to night medication.[8]

## * 1991

– Further evidence of the sedative effects of
lavender oil after inhalation was demonstrated by
a test carried out under standardized experimental
conditions, in which mice were subjected to the
scent of lavender oil. Results showed a significant
decrease in motility, and hyperactivity induced by
a caffeine injection was also reduced almost to
normal.[9]

> It was concluded that the aromatherapeutical use of
> lavender was proven, in that the oil (by its sedative
> effect caused by pharmacological efficacy on the brain)
> could facilitate sleep and minimize stressful situations.[10]

## * 1992

– In a study carried out at the Royal Sussex
County Hospital, patients in intensive and
coronary care were given a 20-minute foot
massage using lavender oil (in an almond oil base)
after receiving physiotherapy. Pain levels,
wakefulness, heart rate and systolic blood-pressure
were measured before and after treatment, then
compared with two control groups – one group
which received a massage using just almond oil,
and another which simply had a 'rest period'.
Results showed that the 'aromatherapy group'
enjoyed the greatest reduction in pain, wakefulness
and blood-pressure – with 91 per cent of patients

experiencing a reduction in heart rate of between 11 and 15 beats per minute.[11]

## * 1993
– A trial conducted with the support of the Bristol Royal Infirmary involved the topical application of two different types of lavender oil – *Lavendula burnatii* (also known as 'lavandin', Sample A) and *L. angustifolia* (Sample B) – to post-cardiotomy patients.[12] The emotional and behavioural stress levels of 28 patients were then evaluated before and after treatment on two consecutive days. The results of this randomized, double-blind study showed that it was possible to move a patient's anxiety level from 'very tense' to 'very relaxed' within 20 minutes by giving the patient a gentle massage using a 5 per cent blend of *L. burnatii*. This method was shown to have a significant relaxant effect and provided a possible alternative to orthodox drug treatment. Key findings were as follows:[13]

- Aromatherapy, using topical application of essential oil, does have measurable therapeutic effects.
- The therapeutic effects are not just due to massage, touch or placebo.
- The choice of essential oils is important.
- It is important to know which lavender is being used.

- One lavender was twice as effective as the other lavender in reducing anxiety.
- Both lavenders greatly aided respiration – essential for post-operative cardiotomies. Twenty out of 24 patients' respirations became slower and deeper.
- More sophisticated research into how aromatherapy works is needed.
- Indiscriminate use of lavender in hospitals should be monitored or avoided.

# Production, Chemical Composition and Quality Control

Although 'true' lavender has been taxonomically classified as *Lavendula vera* de Canolle, *L. officinalis* Chaix, and *L. angustifolia*, it is the latter name which is the correct derivation for the commercially grown aromatic member of the Labiatae family[1]. The original wild lavender (*L. officinalis*) can still be found high on the mountains of southern France where it grows on rocky soil where few other plants can survive. In the heat of July and August the wild lavender was once picked by the local peasants who carried the flowers in bundles on their backs into the valleys for distillation. Some French lavender is still produced from wild plants, but most is now grown on commercially controlled plots or 'communelles', where the lavender essence is graded according to exact analytical specifications and olfactory criteria. Commercial plants are grown from seeds or propagated from cuttings – though an established plant, if well pruned, may last as long as 20 years.

It is generally assumed that the majority of lavender essential oil is still produced in France, but although the French do still grow a lot of lavender, they are not, and have not been, the major producers of the essential oil for many years. The largest producer of lavender oil today is Bulgaria, which produces around 140 tonnes plus per annum, compared to the French who produce about 43 tonnes and falling. Other countries which also produce true lavender oil in quantity are Croatia, Russia, China and Australia, and to a lesser extent, Italy and the US.

At one time, England was also famous for its lavender essence, and lavender production was an important economic aspect of English rural life. The earliest record of lavender being cultivated in England is in an ancient document belonging to Merton Priory from 1301, where there is mention of 'Spikings – 44 quarters', later explained as 'spiking, spike lavender', being grown to raise money for King Edward I. Merton Priory was in the neighbourhood of Mitcham in Surrey – an area which remains famous for its lavender fields even 600 years later! Three hundred acres of lavender were grown in and around Mitcham, in Surrey, during the mid-19th century, and the oil produced there realized six times the price of its French counterpart.

The distillation process was carried out in August when the oil content was at its height, and the fields were harvested by locals who collected the flowers into loose bundles of about one hundredweight, called 'mats' (nowadays most crops are harvested mechanically). At the peak of production in the Mitcham area there were at least six growers supplying the London pharmacists and markets, especially around the area of Buckersbury. Bunches of lavender were also commonly hawked in the London streets – as early as 1805 the text under a print of a lavender seller read:

*'Sixteen bunches a penny, sweet lavender' is the cry that invites in the streets the purchases of this cheap and elegant perfume. The distillers of lavender are supplied wholesale and a considerable quantity is sold in the streets to the middling classes of inhabitants who are fond of placing lavender among the linen yet unwilling to pay for the increased pungency of distillation.*[2]

The earliest forms of extraction were carried out by the process of water distillation. As explained in Chapter 1, the flower heads (not the stalks; using the heads only ensured a top-quality oil) were immersed in a container of water which was then heated. After about half an hour's heating, when the distillate had began to emerge, the fire was dampened down. The aromatic oil was then carried over in a condenser with the water vapour into a copper container, where the distillate separated out into two layers with the volatile oil on top. At the end of six hours the distillation process was complete and the remains of the herb could be cleared away. The Mitcham stills were the largest in Britain and were bigger than the French field stills, with a capacity of between 700 and 1000 gallons. An 1874 survey states that 70 pounds of flowers would yield about one pound of oil – but this appears a very optimistic average!

Although the water distillation technique is still occasionally used in southern France, it was largely supplanted by the more efficient technique of dry steam-distillation at the beginning of the 20th century. In 1906, when this method was introduced, an acre of ground growing about 3,500 plants of English lavender could yield around 15 pounds of pure oil.

By the 1920s the lavender fields had all but disappeared from Mitcham, swamped by suburban development. During the 1930s the centre of lavender growing moved from Surrey to northern Norfolk and centred around the small town of Heacham. Although Norfolk still boasts a high quality essential oil, lavender growing has never again attained the importance it enjoyed in its hey day. Norfolk Lavender still cultivate 100 acres

with several varieties of lavender for the
production of essential oil and dried flowers, but
today the bulk of lavender essential oil used in
Britain is imported for use in traditional toiletries,
air fresheners and perfumes as well as for detergents, waxes and other 'industrial fragrances'. The
highest quality lavender oil, with an ester content
of 50 per cent or more, is reserved for exclusive
perfumes; lavender oil, with an ester content of
around 40 per cent is employed in lavender water
and colognes; while the lower grades (approxi-
mately 30 per cent esters) are used in soap,
detergents, and the like.

*Where* an oil is grown dramatically affects the
balance of its constituents. The same variety of
plant, such as *Lavendula angustifolia*, grown in the
cooler English climate at lower altitudes will
produce a different type of oil or 'chemotype' than
its Mediterranean or Eastern European counterpart. Essential oil qualities also differ from batch
to batch and from crop to crop, even within the
same year – which of course affects the quality of
the fragrance too. It was once thought that high-
altitude lavender produced the best quality oil, but
this is not necessarily the case since factors such as
soil type and other environmental conditions also
play their part.

There are over 150 different constituents in
lavender oil, but the two main ones are *linalool*

and *linalyl acetate* — it is these which give lavender its light, sweetish note. The linalyl acetate (ester) content of lavender oil is also used as a criterion of quality. Typical constituents of lavender oil (*L. angustifolia*) usually fall into the following range:

linalyl acetate 36–51 per cent
linalool 29–46 per cent
lavandulyl acetate 3.4–6.2 per cent
terpinen -4-ol 2.7–6.9 per cent
ocimenes 2.5–10.8 per cent
caryophyllene 2.5–7.6 per cent
1,8-cineole 0.1–2.2 per cent

The setting up of 'communelles' in France has enabled suppliers to offer buyers within the industry large weights of essence of a similar price and quality, but over the years this has also led to a growing trend in France towards the production of 'speciality compositions'. This means that the suppliers 'treat' or 'build up' the primary essence to correspond to different quality levels according to the price that the buyers are willing to pay. Unfortunately, adulteration is all too common, as two of the major constituents — linalool and linalyl acetate — can be produced synthetically at a fraction of the cost. In the 1992 season, for example, official figures proved that the French produced less then 50 tonnes of lavender, yet they still managed to export well in excess of 100 tonnes!

Nowadays, gas chromatography is the main method used for analysing the exact composition of essential oils and for ascertaining their quality. A skilled technician can easily identify a lavender oil cut with synthetic linalool, since there is a sub-component in synthetic linalool (called dihydro-linalool) which does not occur naturally in lavender oil. This trace would show up on a GLC (gas chromatography) machine – where the presence and position of each peak on the graph indicates the amount of each component.

Much of the lavender which is commonly available has been extended/blended in this manner, although oils from Eastern Europe are less likely to have been tampered with, due to these countries' lack of 'technical sophistication'. A high quality pure essential oil of true lavender should be a pale yellow, mobile liquid with a pungent top note which quickly disperses, leaving a soft, fresh, floral and long-lasting aroma. As with tea tree oil, however, recent research has shown that different species and 'chemotypes' of lavender oil have different therapeutic effects, so the 'quality' of an essence in the context of aromatherapy depends largely on its specific use and appropriateness, rather than simply on its aesthetic appeal.

# Summary of the Properties and Applications of Lavender Oil

Lavender oil has often been called the most versatile of all essential oils...but why? By examining its history of use, medical applications and its chemical make-up, it becomes clear that lavender has several diverse areas of activity, being a valuable oil for both physical and psychological complaints. It may be useful, therefore, to divide its principal applications into the following loose categories: skin care; as a soothing remedy/for pain relief; and to help with stress-related conditions. Its secondary uses are also discussed below.

## SKIN CARE

Lavender is an oil with good **antiseptic/ bactericidal, anti-inflammatory** and **cicatrizant** (wound-healing) properties, which makes it an excellent treatment for all types of external injuries or infections. These properties account for why it is such a useful household first-aid remedy for minor cuts, bites, burns and stings. Such applications have been well researched and documented, principally in France.

As a **deodorant** and **antiseborrhoeic** oil, lavender is also a valuable skin care agent and is used for a wide range of common skin conditions such as acne, eczema, seborrhoea and spots. It has been credited with **'rejuvenating'** properties, and since it also has a pleasing floral fragrance, lavender has a long history of traditional use throughout Europe as an ingredient in various types of cosmetic and toiletry preparations, including the famous 'lavender water'.

## SOOTHING REMEDY/ PAIN RELIEF

As a penetrating and soothing **analgesic**, **muscle decontractant** and **antispasmodic** agent, lavender is very valuable for all types of conditions involving spasm or pain such as rheumatism, arthritis, muscular aches and pains, cramp, toothache, earache, period pains or indigestion.

# STRESS-RELATED CONDITIONS

Perhaps of the greatest value, and what makes lavender unique in comparison to other oils such as tea tree, is its pronounced **regulating** effect on the nervous system. Within both the physical and psychological realm lavender is a 'reconciler of opposites', having an essentially **balancing** and **harmonizing** nature. In an age of extremes, it is this quality above all which may account for the strength of the popularity of lavender today! It is also this area of application which is receiving the closest examination in research studies and trials.

Of all essential oils, lavender seems to represent 'the middle way' — being neither 'yin' nor 'yang' in the extreme. This 'neutral' quality may also account for why lavender blends so readily with other essential oils — it also tends to increase the overall effectiveness of a remedy when used in combination with it. In this respect, lavender is a supreme 'adaptogen', i.e. it can have a **restorative** effect in cases of listlessness or weakness, yet has a **calming** effect on those prone to hyperactivity or agitation. This is why it is recommended for what appears to be such a diverse variety of symptoms including shortness of breath, depression and nervous exhaustion as well as palpitations, hysteria and hypertension. In his work with psychiatric patients, Prof Rovesti[1] noted that some essential oils, including lavender, were useful for treating both anxiety and depression or, indeed, a combination of the two:

> It is obviously not possible to define precise limits between the two aromatherapeutic actions of nerve stimulants and nerve sedatives...because of their particular type of physiological action, which Kobert has defined as simultaneously both stimulating and sedative.[2]

This **regulating** action can be seen most clearly with regard to the action of lavender oil on the nervous system as a whole. It is well known that lavender can have either a **tonic** or/and a **sedative** effect on the central nervous system depending on the state of the individual concerned. This makes it one of the most valuable oils for all types of stress-related conditions, where the nervous system can often be both depleted and over-stimulated simultaneously. Stress also depletes the immune system, and can be the cause or the precipitating agent for all types of secondary conditions such as digestive or circulatory problems — a fact which is being increasingly recognized by the orthodox medical establishment today. Lavender is consequently particularly valuable in psychosomatic conditions of this type, where a physical condition is closely related to an underlying psychological state.

Lavender essential oil has also been shown to inhibit both sympathetic and parasympathetic nervous system functioning, depending on which system is dysfunctional. Sympathetic hyper-functioning is triggered more by physical stress, while parasympathetic overactivity is caused more by emotional stress – although both reactions can produce similar symptoms such as muscular cramp, indigestion, spasms or restlessness. By selectively inhibiting either the sympathetic or parasympathetic nervous excess, lavender can assist the body's response to unproductive stress of any kind. Yet lavender will not interfere with the body's response to a productive type of stress, which is a normal and even desirable part of life.

In a similar fashion, lavender can exert either a **cooling** or **warming** effect on the entire system, depending on the temperament and condition of the individual in question. For a person with a hot, acute condition such as a fever or an inflammation, a small amount of lavender will have a **cooling**, effect. On the other hand, for someone suffering from a cold condition such as a chill, muscular cramp or nervous debility, a more generous application of lavender will generate **warmth** and activity, both local and systemic. Thus, by creating an equilibrium within the body, lavender can effect both physical and the psychological changes, thereby enhancing an individual's overall health.[3]

# SECONDARY APPLICATIONS

Lavender has **fungicidal** qualities and is a valuable **prophylactic** agent and **immuno-stimulant**, although these properties are not as pronounced as in the case of tea tree oil. Nevertheless, lavender is a useful **preventative** remedy, acting as a protection against all types of infectious conditions including colds, flu, etc., and may also be used as a treatment for genito-urinary or respiratory infections such as cystitis or bronchitis. In cases of fever, lavender has in addition a **diaphoretic** (sweat-promoting) and **antipyretic** (fever-reducing) effect.

Lavender oil also has many other secondary qualities including its **anti-toxic**, **anti-venomous**, **vermifuge** and **parasiticidal** properties. This makes it a good remedy for all kinds of insect bites and stings. It is also an effective **insecticide** and has been used to repel moths and other insects, such as mosquitoes, for centuries.

*Methods of Use, Safety Data and Storage Precautions*

## METHODS OF USE

### Lavender in the Bath

Add 8–10 drops to the bath water once the bath is full, then relax in the water for at least 10 minutes.

For bathing the feet or hands, add 6–8 drops of lavender oil to a bowl or shallow bath of warm water and soak for 5–10 minutes.

### As a Compress/Poultice

A simple disinfectant compress can be made by dipping a flannel (face-cloth) or piece of cotton wool (cotton ball) in a bowl of water (either steaming hot or ice cold, as required) to which has been added 3–5 drops of lavender oil. A poultice can be made by adding a few drops

of lavender to a clay or kaolin base, and mixing
well.

## Direct/Neat Application

Use the oil direct from the bottle – dabbing with
the fingertips or using a cotton bud (cotton swab)
– to treat cuts, burns, spots, etc.

*Note: Most essential oils should not be used neat on the
skin. Lavender oil is an exception to this rule, however.*

## Gargling and Dental Care

For the treatment of mouth and gum infections,
add 5–10 drops of lavender oil to a glass of warm
water, mix well, then rinse the mouth and/or
gargle.

## Inhalation

Use up to 8 drops on a tissue or handkerchief for
inhalation throughout the day (or onto a pillow for
night use). For respiratory complaints, make a
steam inhalation by adding about 5 drops of
lavender to a bowl of steaming water. Cover your
head with a towel and breathe deeply for about
5–10 minutes with your eyes closed.

## *Massage*

Before being applied to the skin for massage purposes, lavender (like other essential oils) should always be mixed with a light vegetable oil carrier or base such as sweet almond oil, jojoba or grapeseed – although sunflower or soya oil would also suffice. Jojoba oil, being a liquid wax, does not go rancid – otherwise a little wheatgerm oil should be added to the blend to prolong its shelf life. The dilution should be in the region of 2–3 per cent – though sometimes 5 per cent may be used for a concentrated effect, as in the case of local muscular pain, for example.

A rough guideline is to say that 20 drops of essential oil is equivalent to one millilitre, so an easy way of calculating the proportions for general use is to measure the carrier oil in millilitres, then add about half the number of drops of essential oil to give a 2.5 per cent dilution:

| | |
|---|---|
| 100 ml base oil | 50 drops essential oil |
| 50 ml base oil | 25 drops essential oil |
| 1 tbsp (approx. 15 ml) base oil | 7–8 drops essential oil |
| 1 tsp (approx. 5 ml) base oil | 2–3 drops essential oil |

## *Shampoo and Hair Care*

Buy a good, neutral pH value shampoo and add your own lavender to it. To a 100-ml bottle add about 60 drops of lavender oil. An alcohol-based scalp rub can be made by adding 5 ml of lavender to 100 ml of vodka – this can be used to rid the hair of fleas and lice (though it should not be used on irritated skin).

## *Sitz Bath/Douche*

For vaginal and genito-urinary infections, add 6–8 drops of lavender oil to a shallow bath or bowl of warm water and bathe the affected area.

## *Skin Treatments – Creams, Gels, Lotions, Masks and Oils*

The proportions used for mixing skin creams, gels, masks and oils are the same as those for massage purposes – see page 41. For skin care, additional carrier oils such as avocado, hazelnut, borage, peach and apricot kernel can also be included in the blend to suit different skin types.

A light, simple lavender water can be made up using 100 ml distilled water and 25 drops of lavender oil – shake well before use.

## *Vaporization*

There are many vaporizing methods available now
– you can use a terracotta oil burner, an electric
diffuser, or you can simply put a few drops of
lavender oil in a small bowl of hot water placed
on a radiator or any other source of heat. This
method is particularly useful for disinfecting a sick
room and preventing the spread of contagious
illness. Lavender may also be used to repel insects
in this manner.

## *Other Measures*

Many common conditions benefit from combin-
ing aromatherapy with other approaches such as
herbal medicine, acupuncture, counselling, dietary
changes and exercise. Essential oils and allopathic
medicines can also complement one another –
check with a qualified herbalist or aromatherapy
practitioner for further advice.

## SAFETY DATA

Lavender is non-toxic, non-irritating and non-
sensitizing. It is one of the safest essential oils,
with low toxicity levels and no contra-indications.
  Babies, young children and pregnant women

should take special care using all essential oils, because of their concentration. Despite lavender's low toxicity level, it is advisable not to use it neat for the treatment of children under 18 months of age – and always dilute for use during pregnancy to half the usual recommended amount.

*Note: ESSENTIAL OILS SHOULD NOT BE TAKEN INTERNALLY!*

## STORAGE

For storage purposes lavender oil should be kept in an airtight dark-glass container, away from light and heat and well out of the reach of children or pets. The pure oil can also interact with certain plastics – plastic containers are therefore best avoided.

IT IS VERY IMPORTANT TO OBTAIN LAVENDER FROM A REPUTABLE SOURCE TO ENSURE A SAFE AND EFFECTIVE THERAPEUTIC RESULT!

# PART II

# A–Z of Health Care Applications

## ABSCESS/BOIL (FURUNCLE)

An abscess or boil is a localized painful swelling and inflammation of the skin, due to an infection of a sebaceous gland.

Abscesses usually appear when the body is run-down or stressed, at times of hormonal upheaval or as the result of a blood disorder. Whatever the cause, the presence of an abscess or boil indicates that the system is in need of purification: Avoid stimulants, eat lots of fresh fruit and vegetables and drink plenty of water or herb teas (especially those which purify the blood).

- Never wait for the boil or abscess to burst — treat as soon as it begins to appear by dabbing with neat lavender oil. Repeat 2 or 3 times a day.
- If the boil/abscess has already formed, apply a warm poultice of clay containing 3–4 drops

lavender oil. Leave for half an hour to draw
the liquid/pus, then bathe gently with water.
Alternatively, apply a warm flannel (face-cloth)
which has been soaked in a lavender solution,
then dab the boil with neat lavender oil.
Repeat 2 or 3 times a day.

- If the boil/abscess is severe, cover with a
  gauze soaked in lavender oil for 12 hours. If
  there is still no improvement, seek medical
  advice.
- Add 8–10 drops of lavender oil to the bath
  water as a general disinfectant measure.
- Tea tree oil may be used in the same manner (or
  in combination with lavender).

## ACNE (AND SPOTS)

This unsightly skin condition is caused by an
overactivity of the sebaceous glands, and is
especially common during adolescence, the
menopause and at times of hormonal upheaval,
such as before or during menstruation.

A very greasy, congested skin results in a rough
surface texture, enlarged pores, spots, pimples and
blackheads. The condition can be exacerbated
further by a poor diet, too little exercise, lack of
hygiene, stress and other emotional factors. Scrupulous attention to hygiene prevents the condition
spreading.

One woman had suffered for a long time

with an oily skin and blackheads, and has used all kinds of creams to no avail.

> *To treat the condition I massaged her face with a [thin, non-greasy] lotion to which I added lavender, geranium and bergamot...I was surprised at how dramatically effective this treatment was. The pores closed up within a short time...and remained closed for a whole week.*[1]

- Apply neat lavender oil to individual spots night and morning using a cotton bud (cotton swab).
- Make up a lavender water using 100 ml distilled water and 25 drops of lavender oil. Shake well before use and bathe the face (and other affected areas) night and morning.
- Make up a 5 per cent non-oily lavender cream or gel (see instructions page 42) to apply as a cleansing/moisturizing ointment.
- Add 8–10 drops of lavender oil to the bath water – this also acts as a facial steam.
- Have a facial sauna 3 or 4 times a week using 3–5 drops of lavender (see page 40).
- Other oils of benefit: tea tree, geranium and bergamot (bergapten-free) – best used in combination with lavender.

## ALOPECIA/BALDNESS
– *see* **Hair Care**

## ANXIETY

Anxiety is one of the most common stress-related conditions encountered today, and is characterized by symptoms such as high blood-pressure, insomnia, palpitations or irritability. If the state of anxiety is allowed to persist over a prolonged period, it can lead to secondary, more serious complaints such as stomach ulcers or heart failure.

The value of lavender oil in helping to counter the effects of anxiety within a clinical context has been confirmed by several scientists including Dr Valnet and Professor Rovesti[2]. The effects of lavender on brainwave patterns has also been researched in recent years. In Japan, Dr Sugano has shown that the scent of lavender increases both alpha brainwave activity (associated with a relaxed mental state) and cerebral blood circulation, while Prof. Torii of Tokyo University includes lavender among those oils having a sedative effect on the central nervous system, based on EEG material.[3] As a result, lavender is being used increasingly in hospital wards today as a massage oil or airborne fragrance to help dispel anxiety, calm the mind and increase general feelings of well-being (see pages 21–5).

* Add 8–10 drops to a warm evening bath to relieve insomnia, restlessness, anxiety, nervous tension or an overactive mind.

- Receiving a regular professional massage using a blend of suitable oils can dramatically reduce anxiety levels. For self-treatment blend 2–3 drops of lavender with 1 tsp sweet almond oil and massage into the hands and the soles of the feet.
- For a soothing room fragrance, use lavender oil in a vaporizer, or put a few drops on a hankie for inhalation throughout the day.
- Other measures: yoga, meditation and psychotherapy. Other essential oils of benefit include bergamot, neroli, ylang ylang and rose.

*See also* **Depression, Insomnia, Stress**

### ARTHRITIS (AND GOUT)

There are several different kinds of arthritis – but all signify the body's inability to eliminate toxic waste efficiently. This causes excess uric acid to be deposited as crystals in the spaces between the joints. The two most common forms are *rheumatoid arthritis*, which can affect all age groups, and *osteoarthritis*, which usually occurs in the elderly. Both are forms of joint distress which can result in pain, inflammation and sometimes deformity.

Gout usually affects the joints of the toes, but also sometimes the fingers.

Stress, emotional conflict, lack of exercise and

poor diet all contribute to these conditions. Aromatic baths and massage can help eliminate the toxic waste, as well as provide relief from pain. Lavender oil is particularly recommended for children suffering from these conditions, because of its relative mildness.

> *I applied a cool compress of lavender, juniper and rosemary and wrapped her knee in a towel. The compress was repeated again after 15 minutes...she was delighted with the results which were relief from pain and increased mobility to the joint.*[1]

- Make a massage oil by mixing 30 drops of lavender oil with 50 ml of a vegetable carrier oil. Very gently, apply twice daily.
- Add 8–10 drops of lavender oil to the bath water for pain relief.
- To ease inflammation, apply a cold compress using clay (or a flannel or face-cloth) to which has been added a few drops of lavender oil.
- *Note:* There are several other oils which are of great benefit in arthritis and are best used in combination: *for detoxifying* – cypress, fennel, juniper, lemon and tea tree; *for inflammation* – chamomile and marjoram; and *for stimulating greater mobility* – pine, rosemary and ginger.

## ASTHMA

Asthma, characterized by wheezing and shortness of breath, commonly appears during early childhood and often ceases at puberty. It usually runs in families and, like many allergic conditions, an attack can be brought on by a number of different factors including diet; contact with allergens such as dust, polish, hairspray or feathers; climatic conditions, especially damp; strenuous exercise; and/or underlying emotional issues.

Many things can be done to alleviate asthma, if the cause of the attack and the pattern of the illness can be identified. As a relaxant and antispasmodic oil, lavender is very helpful for asthma especially when combined with massage. Used as a preventative measure it can keep attacks from occurring so frequently.

One case history shows the benefits of using lavender on a regular basis for massage, baths and inhalation:

*Jodie had a history of eczema from birth to about 6 or 7 years old and thereafter suffered asthma attacks and coughs on a regular basis...Her summers were made miserable by severe hay fever and in previous years she took Triluden on the advice of the school nurse...[after being treated with lavender oil in regular baths, inhalations and as a massage oil consisting of 50 ml sweet almond oil, 9 drops lavender, 3 drops geranium and a little rose oil] despite a two-week camping holiday Jodie did not have to take any Triluden over the summer. Only one asthma attack was experienced...Her parents were really pleased and have now purchased an infuser and some lavender for use in the home.*[5]

- Mix 7–8 drops of lavender with 1 tbs sweet almond oil and massage the back in long sweeping movements, starting at the base of the spine, up over the shoulders, then down the sides of the body.
- Put a few drops of lavender on a tissue for inhalation throughout the day, especially at the onset of an attack.
- Use lavender in vaporizers and in the bath at home as a general precautionary measure.
- Other oils of benefit: frankincense, rose, geranium and chamomile.

**BABIES**
– *see* **Children's Ailments**

**BRONCHITIS**
– *see* **Infectious Illnesses**

**BRUISES/BUMPS**
A bruise indicates that the tissue is damaged beneath the skin's surface as a result of a bump or

pressure to that area. Applying lavender oil reduces inflammation, heals cell tissues and speeds up the healing process.

* Apply a cold compress to ease inflammation, then dab a drop or two of neat lavender oil onto the affected area.
* Arnica ointment and tea tree oil are also very useful bruise remedies.

**BURNS**

Burns can be caused by dry heat or moist heat (scalds), and are often very painful. Minor burns respond extremely well to treatment with essential oils as they reduce the pain, prevent blistering or infection and promote healing.

*Note:* Severe burns, especially if accompanied by shock, require immediate medical attention.

Used by the French in wartime; lavender oil is increasingly being employed for treating burns in hospitals within the UK.

> *Wide superficial burn on the outside of the left thigh caused by mustard gas. Burned 8th September in the Aisne. Since 2nd December, small, ulcerated, excoriated, bloody spots have appeared. Application of lavender from day one and normal dressing. Healed 31st December.*[6]

- Immediately put the affected area under the cold tap for 5 minutes, then apply neat lavender oil to the site of the burn. Continue to apply neat at least 3 times a day until the skin has healed.
- Alternatively, apply a water-based gel to which 5–10 per cent lavender oil has been added.
- Other measures: tea tree essential oil is also a very effective burn remedy when used in the same manner as recommended for lavender oil.

**CARBUNCLES**

A carbuncle is a collection of boils caused by *staphyloccus aureaus* – characterized by a painful node and covered with tight red skin that later becomes thick and discharges pus. Carbuncles are commonly found on the upper back, nape of the neck or the buttocks.

- Keep the area clean and apply neat lavender oil to the site of the problem 3 times a day.
- Add 8–10 drops of lavender to the bath water as a disinfectant measure.
- Tea tree oil can be used in this same manner, or in combination with lavender oil.

**CHICKENPOX**

Chickenpox is a highly contagious viral infection – common during childhood – which is caused by the *herpes zoster* virus. A fever develops and itchy spots appear in crops, progressing to blisters and then to crusts. Zona (shingles) is another condition caused by this virus.

Chickenpox can be accompanied by severe pain, usually before the rash appears, and there may be a fever. It is particularly dangerous for adults, as it is accompanied by a high temperature and pain.

- Use lavender in vaporizers throughout the duration of the illness.
- Soak frequently in tepid water for 10–15 minutes at a time, every few hours if possible. For babies dissolve 2 drops of tea tree and 1 drop of lavender (or chamomile) in 1 tsp of alcohol; for use in the bath for children dissolve 3 drops of tea tree and 2 drops of lavender (or chamomile) in 1 tsp alcohol; for adults dissolve 5 drops tea tree and 5 drops of lavender (or chamomile) in 1 tsp alcohol.
- Dissolve 25 (15 for children) drops of tea tree and 10 (5 for children) drops each of lavender and chamomile in one dessertspoon of alcohol, then mix with 50 ml rosewater and 50 ml witchhazel. Shake well before using – apply frequently to spots using a cotton wool or gauze pad.

    *Note:* this treatment is not suitable for young babies.

- Other measures: a handful of colloidal oatmeal (available from most chemists) may also be added to the bath water to soothe itching and encourage healing. Tea tree is the most valuable oil for chickenpox, applied in the same fashion as lavender, or in combination.

*See also* **Herpes**

## CHILDBIRTH
– *see* **Pregnancy and Childbirth**

## CHILDREN'S AILMENTS
Due to its low toxicity level, lavender is especially suited to the treatment of childhood complaints such as colic, tummy ache, cuts, stings and sores. Lavender is also one of the few essential oils which can be used safely for young children and for a variety of common complaints. Since most children like the smell of lavender, it is also a good choice for bathtime, in a massage oil or as a vaporizer in a child's room.

Babies and infants respond especially well to natural healing methods, but their extra sensitivity must be taken into account. Do not attempt to substitute a home remedy for professional treatment if it is needed. Amounts used should accord with the age of the child:

| | |
|---|---|
| Babies (0–12 months) | 1 drop of lavender diluted in 1 tsp carrier oil for massage or bathing |
| Infants (1–5 years) | 2–3 drops of lavender diluted in 1 tsp carrier oil for massage or bathing |
| Children (6–12 years) | 5–6 drops for bathing, or diluted in 1 tbs carrier oil for massage |
| Teenagers (over 12 years) | use as for adults |

- Nappy (diaper) rash in babies and infants can be prevented by regular bathing using 1 drop of lavender diluted in 1 tsp carrier oil. If nappy rash does occur, add 1 drop each of lavender and tea tree to a non-greasy baby cream.
- Restlessness, hyperactivity and insomnia in babies, infants and older children can be alleviated by the use of lavender in the bath or for massage as directed above. Alternatively use a vaporizer in the bedroom (ensure it is out of reach), or put a drop or two of oil on the pillow or on the child's pyjamas or nightie.
- Tummy ache or colic in babies, infants and older children can be eased by mixing 1–3

drops of lavender in 1 tsp carrier oil and
gently massaging the lower back or stomach in
a clockwise direction.

- Teething pain in babies and infants can be
  relieved by mixing 1 drop of lavender in 1 tsp
  of carrier oil and massaging onto the outer
  cheek.
- Cradle cap is an unsightly scalp condition
  which affects very young babies, especially the
  newborn. A thick, yellowish crust develops on
  the scalp and there is often scaling behind the
  ears. Mix fresh for each treatment 5 drops of
  lavender oil with 1 dessertspoon of slightly
  warmed olive oil and rub this gently into the
  scalp. Leave for 5–10 minutes then wash out
  using lavender shampoo (the scalp may remain
  slightly oily after treatment). Take care to
  avoid the eyes while rinsing. Repeat daily
  initially, then continue using lavender
  shampoo as part of the baby's normal routine
  to prevent a recurrence. (Tea tree oil is also
  effective for cradle cap when used in the same
  fashion.)
- For cuts, spots, insect bites and other skin
  blemishes for infants over 1 year old, apply
  1 drop of neat lavender.
- Chamomile is a also a very useful children's
  remedy which can be used in the same way as
  lavender, or in combination with it.

- *Note:* ALL ESSENTIAL OILS, INCLUDING LAVENDER, SHOULD BE KEPT WELL OUT OF THE REACH OF CHILDREN.

**COLDS**
– *see* **Infectious Illnesses**

**COLD SORES**
– *see* **Herpes**

**CRACKED SKIN**
Dry, cracked skin on the feet and hands is a common problem, especially during the winter months. In severe cases it can be painful, especially in association with frostbite or skin complaints such as psoriasis.

- Mix 3 drops of lavender with 1 tsp wheatgerm oil (or a thick moisturizing cream) and massage well into the affected area night and morning. Continue until the condition improves.
- Other measures: benzoin, myrrh, tea tree and patchouli are also useful essential oils for cracked skin when used individually or in combination and applied as you would lavender oil.

*See also* **Skin Care**

## CUTS/WOUNDS

Small cuts and scratches are among the most common household injuries, especially where young children are concerned. Lavender is an excellent first-aid remedy for all sorts of skin abrasions or wounds due to its excellent antiseptic and wound-healing properties. It is so gentle that it does not sting the exposed raw skin, and it acts as a mild anaesthetic and encourages a rich flow of blood to the damaged area. It also prevents scarring:

> *I grabbed the lavender oil and poured it over the wound. Without pain of any description, I promise you that I stood and watched the gaping hole close before my eyes...By evening I had a small scar that looked rather like a wrinkle, and the following morning even the wrinkle had disappeared.*[7]

Even stubborn sores or wounds will often respond to lavender:

> *Infected sore on the posterior side of the instep, dating back 18 days. All the usual methods had been tried: dry and wet dressings, ointments and powders. One application of lavender. Twenty-four hours later, the sore was dry and healed.*[8]

- Clean the area thoroughly with water, then dab on a few drops of pure lavender oil. Apply a plaster (adhesive bandage) if required.

Continue to apply the lavender oil neat several times a day until the skin has healed.
- Other measures: pure tea tree oil can be used as an alternative.

## CYSTITIS/URETHRITIS

Cystitis is a bacterial infection of the bladder, more common among women than men. It is characterized by a frequent need to urinate, a painful burning sensation while passing water (which is often cloudy) and sometimes feverishness. Many attacks of cystitis start as urethritis – an infection of the urethra.

*Note:* If symptoms do not improve within a few days, or if there is blood or pus in the urine, seek professional help immediately.

- Make up a solution using 10 drops of lavender oil in half a litre of cooled boiled water. Using a piece of soaked cotton wool (a cotton ball), swab the opening of the urethra frequently (if possible, after each time you pass water).
- Add 8–10 drops to the bath water – it is beneficial to bathe frequently using bactericidal oils as a general disinfectant and preventative measure.
- Make up a massage oil using 3 drops of lavender oil in 1 tsp light carrier oil (such as jojoba or

grapeseed) and rub gently into the lower
abdomen and back. Repeat at least twice daily.
• Other measures: drink plenty of water or
herbal teas; avoid tight-fitting clothes and nylon
underwear; take a course of garlic capsules;
bergamot, tea tree, chamomile and sandalwood
essential oils are also of benefit when used as
you would lavender oil.

## DEPRESSION

Depression can take many forms: it is often
associated with a lack of energy and listlessness but
it can also be accompanied by restlessness or
agitation — or by a combination of both lethargy
and excitement.

Lavender has long been used to help alleviate
depression, but is especially valuable where there
is a tendency towards 'mood swings', due to its
regulating or stabilizing nature. Essential oils such
as lavender are also very beneficial when coping
with difficult life situations involving emotions
such as grief, loss or fear. One doctor who
recognizes the value of aromatics in this field
describes her own reasons for using aromatherapy
after the death of her mother:

*I didn't want tranquillizers and didn't feel anti-*
*depressants were needed as mine was a perfectly normal*
*reaction to the stress I was living through. I didn't*

*want to take alcohol and yet craved relief from what I was experiencing. I knew these pharmacological treatments did not work for real-life situations of stress. They might work for people with neurotic problems, or those in a state of clinical depression, but that's a different thing. I didn't have any of those symptoms...A combination of massage and essential oils (especially lavender) is more powerful than either one alone, and [makes for] a valuable form of relaxation therapy.*[9]

- Add 8–10 drops of lavender oil to the bath – best used in combination with other anti-depressant oils such as jasmine, rose, neroli or bergamot.
- Receiving a regular professional massage using a blend of anti-depressant oils including lavender can help encourage relaxation and feelings of self-worth and well-being. Research has shown that the 'synergistic' combination of smell and touch can have a profoundly nourishing and comforting effect on the psyche.
- For an uplifting/soothing room fragrance, use lavender oil in a vaporizer, or put a few drops on a hankie for inhalation throughout the day.
- Other measures: yoga, meditation and psychotherapy/counselling. Other essential oils of benefit include bergamot, neroli, jasmine and rose.

*See also* **Anxiety, Stress**

## DERMATITIS/ECZEMA

Dermatitis and eczema are general terms used to describe a variety of inflamed or irritated skin conditions characterized by redness, flaky skin, rashes and itching, which in turn can lead to blisters, weepy sores and scabs.

The cause of the problem can vary – though many forms of dermatitis are associated with hereditary allergic tendencies, especially to certain foods (notably dairy or wheat products). Another form, known as contact dermatitis, is the result of the skin's hypersensitivity to an external irritant such as a type of detergent or cosmetic, or to dust, wool or some other substance. It is often very difficult to identify the cause, because the reaction may appear some time after the initial contact, or the skin may suddenly react adversely to a familiar substance. In all cases, however, mental stress or other emotional factors tend to aggravate or trigger an attack.

*Note:* It may be necessary to experiment with different essential oils and types of treatment due to the individual nature of these types of skin problems.

- Apply pure lavender oil to the affected area.
- For larger areas, make up a 1 per cent lavender gel or non-oily cream (see instructions page

42) and apply to the affected area twice daily.

- Add 8–10 drops of lavender oil to the bath water.
- Other measures: try to identify and remove causes of irritation; assess and improve the emotional environment if possible; the essential oils of chamomile, tea tree, melissa, neroli and bergamot (bergapten-free) are also beneficial for skin complaints of this type – either used individually or in combination, employed in the bath or in creams/gels.

## DISINFECTANT USES

Lavender has good antimicrobial properties and makes an excellent disinfectant agent since it does not irritate the skin and has a pleasing floral fragrance. During the Second World War, every English home with a lavender bush was asked to harvest the flowers and take them to the local medical supplies unit for use as an antiseptic! At this time it was also used to wipe down floors and bench surfaces in field hospitals and operating theatres, as well as for swabbing wounds.

- Disinfecting clothes, nappies (diapers), etc.: for hand washing, add up to 50 drops of lavender oil to half a litre of warm water; otherwise add up to 50 drops to a liquid detergent before putting it into the washing machine.

- For washing floors, surfaces, etc.: add up
  to 50 drops to a bucket or bowl of water
  and stir well before mopping or wiping
  surfaces.
- For cleaning cuts, wounds, etc.: add a few
  drops of neat lavender to a small bowl of
  cooled boiled water and swab the damaged
  area using a cotton wool or gauze pad.
- Disinfecting sickrooms, bathrooms, workplaces,
  etc.: diffuse lavender into the air – for various
  methods see page 43.
- Several other essential oils are also valuable
  disinfectants – notably tea tree but also lemon
  and eucalyptus.

## DIZZINESS
– *see* **Shock/Vertigo**

## DYSPEPSIA (INDIGESTION) AND FLATULENCE
Dyspepsia or indigestion is a common complaint
among both children and adults. As a carminative
and antispasmodic agent, lavender is especially
valuable for all types of digestive disorders where
there is a strong nervous or emotional element
involved...in the *British Herbal Pharmacopoeia*,
lavender is indicated specifically for 'depressive
states associated with digestive dysfunction'.

- Mix 3 drops of lavender in 1 tsp of carrier oil

and massage the tummy gently in a clockwise
direction.
* Other measures: chamomile or peppermint oil
are also helpful, used in combination;
chamomile, peppermint or fennel herb tea,
with a little honey, are also beneficial.

*See also* **Stress**

**EARACHE**
Earache often accompanies mild respiratory
complaints such as sinusitis or a cold, and in some
cases can lead to a more serious infection. If there
is a high temperature, or if pain is severe or
persistent, seek professional advice immediately.

* Massage gently around the painful area using
3 drops of lavender diluted in 1 tsp carrier oil.
* Soak a cotton wool ball in 1 tsp warm olive or
almond oil to which 3 drops of lavender have
been added, and insert gently into the outer
ear.
* *Note:* this should only be done after a medical
examination to ensure the ear drum is not
perforated.
* Additional measures: keep warm, especially the
area of the affected ear; chamomile oil can be
used in the same way as lavender.

**ECZEMA**
– *see* **Dermatitis**

**EPILEPSY**
Epilepsy is the most common serious neurological disorder: up to 5 per cent of the population will have at least one epileptic fit during their lifetime. Although aromatherapy cannot be said to be a cure for epilepsy, if used in conjunction with conventional therapy it can be a very valuable aid for many sufferers.

> With Joan, it was clear that her fear of the attack was actually reinforcing it. Using lavender as her chosen oil, she has developed a good counter-measure response for whenever she feels her seizures start...she has now become seizure-free.[10]

- Use in baths, vaporizers and for massage.
- Particularly, apply lavender to a handkerchief and sniff it at the onset of a seizure.
- Additional measures: Ylang ylang, chamomile and bergamot have been found to be effective in some cases.

**FATIGUE**
Lavender has long been used as a nerve tonic in cases of debility or nervous exhaustion, indeed lavender water was originally made as a reviving

perfume for 'languor and weakness of the nerves, lowness of spirits, faintings, etc'. According to Mrs Grieve, lavender essential oil is also 'admirably restorative' and 'a few drops of the essence of lavender in a hot footbath has a marked influence in relieving fatigue'.[11]

- Add 8–10 drops to the bath, or footbath, as a reviving 'pick-me-up'.
- Simply inhaling lavender from a tissue in the same fashion as you would 'smelling salts' can help counteract feelings of weakness, dizziness or nervous weakness.
- Lavender also acts as a tonic to the nervous system when used in massage oils, baths, inhalations, etc.

**FLATULENCE**
– *see* **Dyspepsia**

**FLU**
– *see* **Infectious Illnesses**

**GENITAL HERPES**
– *see* **Herpes**

**HAIR CARE**
Lavender oil makes an excellent conditioning treatment for the hair due to its pleasing scent,

gentle action and powerful antiseptic properties. It helps to regulate the activity of the sebaceous glands, cleanses the scalp of bacterial infection and helps disperse dead skin cells. It has the reputation of 'sorting knots and tangles' and also encourages hair growth.

> Dr Marchand has studied the question of hair loss and his studies have led to the conclusion that pure lavender essence used as a scalp massage reduces hair loss and encourages regrowth.[12]

By making the hair more healthy and manageable, lavender oil benefits all hair types including dry hair, greasy hair and itchy scalp conditions.

- Choose a mild or pH neutral shampoo which does not strip the hair of its protective acid mantle, then add between 1 and 3 per cent of lavender oil (about 20–60 drops per 100 ml of mild shampoo – or 2–3 drops of lavender oil to 1 tsp of shampoo). Shampoo daily or according to your usual routine – this treatment is good for all hair types.
- Lavender oil can also be added to a conditioning lotion in the same manner (2 per cent), or a few drops can be put in the final rinse water.
- For a hair conditioner to encourage hair growth and to treat baldness (alopecia): mix

25 drops of lavender oil with 50 ml of slightly warmed jojoba or coconut oil, massage thoroughly into scalp. Wrap hair in a warm towel and leave for an hour if possible. Wash out, using lavender shampoo – apply the shampoo first before the water, otherwise the hair will remain oily. Repeat once a week. (Alternatively, a few drops of lavender oil can be added to a natural conditioning lotion or wax – or rubbed neat into the scalp).

• A good final rinse for all hair types is to add 5 drops of lavender and 1 tbsp of cider vinegar to the final rinse water. This will help to remove detergent residue and restore the acid equilibrium of the scalp.

• Other essential oils which are excellent for hair care include tea tree, rosemary, chamomile and West Indian bay.

*See also* **Children's Ailments (Cradle Cap), Lice**

### HEADACHES

Headaches can be caused by a number of different factors – sinus congestion, nervous stress, eye strain, too much sun or too much alcohol!

Lavender is particularly indicated for tension headaches and to prevent sunstroke. At one time it was common for farmers to keep a sprig of lavender under their hat...and it was 'a notable fact that they never suffered from headaches despite working in the bright sunshine for many hours'.[13]

• Inhale lavender oil from a tissue, or apply neat to the temples or on a cold compress to the forehead or back of the neck.
• Headaches brought on by tension or stress can also be eased by a firm neck and shoulder massage using 3 drops of lavender in 1 tsp carrier oil.

*See also* **Stress**

**HERPES**
Cold sores, usually found on the lips or face, are caused by the virus *herpes simplex I*. The condition is infectious and can be spread to other parts of the body or to other people quite easily. Some people are particularly prone to cold sores, especially when they are run down or have suffered exposure to cold wind or hot sunshine.

Genital herpes is an infection transmitted by sexual contact and caused by the virus *herpes simplex II*. The first attack is generally the worst; the skin of the genital region becomes red and itchy and then erupts into small, very painful blisters which can last for several weeks. This tends to be followed by recurrent attacks which take a milder form, often precipitated by stress, sexual activity or another infection; these subsequent attacks usually last only a few days. Nevertheless, genital herpes remains a very distressing condition that does not respond to standard antibiotic treatment (like cold sores, which also do not respond to antibiotics).

- Use neat lavender oil to dab any blisters or sores as soon as they begin to develop – check for skin sensitivity first! Repeat frequently over a period of several days, or until the condition has cleared.
- In the case of genital herpes, at the very first sign of infection make a concentrated solution by mixing 30 drops of lavender oil with about 1 litre of warm water – shake or stir well before use. Use this solution to douche or wash the genital area frequently to soothe irritation and prevent the infection from developing. In addition, all sexual partners should also undergo treatment to avoid re-infection; abstain from sexual contact for at least a week during the treatment.
- *Note:* Although it is normal to experience a temporary warm sensation, discontinue this treatment if irritation occurs.
- Add 8–10 drops to the bath water as a general disinfectant measure.

• Other measures: take vitamin C tablets; bergamot (bergapten-free) oil and especially tea tree oil are also beneficial for treating herpes when applied in the same manner as lavender.

*See also* **Chicken Pox**

**HIGH BLOOD-PRESSURE (HYPERTENSION)**
Many people suffer from high blood-pressure these days, for it is a common side-effect of the fast pace of 20th-century life. Stress, poor diet, too much alcohol and arteriosclerosis (the thickening and hardening of the arterial walls) can all contribute to this condition, which in the long term may lead to a serious kidney disease or heart failure. It is therefore vital to reduce blood-pressure levels as soon as possible, and one's diet, lifestyle, ambitions, etc. often need to be reassessed. Lavender is a valuable treatment for high blood-pressure according to several accounts:

> *In 1990, Nikolaevskii examined the effect of lavender oil volatiles [volatile oils] on atherosclerosis in rabbits. Although they found that there was no reduction of the cholesterol in the blood, there was reported reduction of cholesterol in the aorta thereby causing a reduced atherosclerotic plaque deposition.*[14]

Aromatherapy massage has also been found to be

especially effective in implementing change in this field:

> Long-term studies in a London teaching hospital have shown that massage effectively reduces high blood-pressure, and that this effect persists for a long time. When massage is given regularly, the effects are even more striking, and blood-pressure may be lowered for several days after a massage. The most important oils to use in these circumstances are Lavender, Marjoram and Ylang ylang.[15]

- If possible, put aside some time each week to have a regular professional massage using a blend of relaxing oils including lavender. Self-massage or massage between partners or friends is also valuable.
- Add 8–10 drops of lavender oil to the bath – or in combination with other relaxing oils such as ylang ylang, chamomile or marjoram.
- Use lavender oil in a vaporizer at home or in the office on a regular basis, or put a few drops on a hankie for inhalation throughout the day.
- Other measures: yoga, meditation and psychotherapy/counselling; reduce intake of stimulants including tea, coffee and alcohol.

*See also* **Anxiety, Stress**

**HYPERTENSION**
– *see* **High Blood-pressure**

**IMMUNE SYSTEM (TO STRENGTHEN)**
Many essential oils, including lavender (but
particularly tea tree oil) stimulate the immune
system and can assist the body in resisting as well
as combating infection:

1. by directly opposing the threatening micro-
   organisms
2. by stimulating and increasing the activity of the
   organs and cells involved
3. by building up resistance and promoting the
   immune system as a whole.

   *People who use essential oils all the time, as part of*
   *their daily bathing, skin care and household routines,*
   *mostly have a high level of resistance to illness,*
   *'catching' fewer colds, etc. than average and recovering*
   *quickly if they do.*[16]

• To help build up resistance levels, take a bath
  at least twice a week using 8–10 drops of
  lavender (or tea tree) oil in the water.
• To strengthen the immune system, have a
  massage once a week using a 2.5 per cent
  lavender (or tea tree) oil blend (see
  instructions page 41). If this is not possible,

make up a 5 per cent concentrated massage oil blend and rub this firmly into the palms of the hands and soles of the feet once a day.
- Use lavender and other essential oils (particularly tea tree) as room fragrances on an everyday basis.
- Other measures: a course of garlic capsules, vitamin E and vitamin C are also indicated.

## IMPETIGO

This highly infectious skin disease which mainly affects children is usually caused by an invasion of the *streptococcus* or *staphylococcus* bacteria. Inflamed patches or spots appear, usually on the face, scalp and neck, but sometimes on the hands and knees – which blister and then crust over.

The bactericidal action of lavender makes it very effective in treating this contagious skin condition. Strict hygiene is also essential to prevent the condition from spreading to other parts of the body – or to other people.

- Apply pure lavender oil to affected areas, using the tip of the finger or a cotton bud (swab). Repeat twice a day.
- Add 10 drops (no more than 5 for children) to the bath water as a disinfectant measure.
- Tea tree is also an effective remedy, alone or in combination with lavender.

INDIGESTION
– see **Dyspepsia**

**INFECTIOUS ILLNESSES**
Lavender is a useful remedy to have at hand during
an infectious illness such as bronchitis, flu or the
common cold, due to its ability to ease both
physical and psychological discomfort and because
of its balancing nature or 'two-way effect':

> *Possibly the best instance in which lavender's two-way
> effect is put to use simultaneously is at the onset of an
> infection such as fever, sore throat, headache, aches
> and pains and unrest. In this condition lavender's
> predominating calming actions – anti-inflammatory,
> analgesic, antipyretic and nervous system sedative –
> will relieve symptoms resulting from the individual's
> response to the infection. However, its mainly
> stimulating actions – diaphoretic, anti-infective and
> antiseptic – will directly address the source of the
> condition – the infection itself.*[17]

• Use lavender in vaporizers throughout the
  duration of the illness, or add a few drops to a
  hankie for inhalation throughout the day, and
  to the pillow for night use.
• Take a daily hot bath adding 8–10 drops of
  lavender to the water – this soothes aching
  limbs and also acts as a kind of steam
  inhalation.

- For a sore throat, add 5–10 drops of lavender to a glass of warm water, mix well and gargle. Repeat at least 2 or 3 times a day.
- Other measures: take a course of garlic capsules and vitamin C tablets. Tea tree or eucalyptus are excellent anti-infectious agents; marjoram or chamomile oil can also be used in baths to soothe aching limbs and encourage restful sleep.

## INSECT BITES/STINGS

Lavender oil has long been used for the treatment of a variety of insect bites and stings – at one time it was even used to treat snake bite!

> In the Alps, if their dogs are bitten by adders, huntsmen will get lavender, crush it and rub it on the bites. The venom is neutralized immediately.[18]

Lavender has also been found to bring fast relief from the bites of mosquitoes, fleas and horseflies – as well as wasp and bee stings! Dabbed directly onto the bite it not only soothes itching and relieves pain but also prevents any infection from developing further due to scratching – especially among children.

Lavender oil also makes an excellent insect repellent – and has been used for centuries to protect clothes and linen from moths.

- To treat bites and stings apply neat lavender oil to the affected area – repeat every 4 hours or as required.
- As a preventative measure, lavender oil can be applied neat to exposed skin; to clothing such as socks, scarves, etc.; or diluted in a light vegetable oil base for application to larger areas.
- To keep insects out of the house, apply lavender to hanging ribbons or use a vaporizer.
- Other measures: there are several oils with insect-repellent properties, the most useful being tea tree, citronella, lemongrass, eucalyptus or atlas cedarwood – or a combination of these.

## INSOMNIA

Sleeplessness or insomnia is another common stress-related complaint that everyone suffers from at some time in life – whether it is before an exam, after an exhilarating experience, or simply due to an inability to switch off after a hard day's work.

Lavender is a traditional remedy for insomnia – this is why lavender pillows and lavender-scented linen were once so popular – the scent alone encourages a restful night's sleep. An old lavender remedy for 'they that may not sleep' runs as follows:

> *...seep this herb in water and let him soak his feet to the ankles at bedtime and bind it on the temples, and he shall sleep well by the Grace of God.*[19]

- For a quick (modern) home treatment, massage a few drops of neat lavender oil into the soles of the feet before retiring. This will quickly be absorbed through the skin into the bloodstream and act as a natural sedative.
- To encourage relaxation or a restful night (also excellent during pregnancy and for children), use the vaporized oil in the bedroom, or put a few drops on the pillow or on pyjamas. Sheets scented with lavender oil also help induce sleep.
- Put 8–10 drops of lavender in a warm bath before retiring for the night, and relax for at least 10 minutes in the aromatic vapours.
- A regular professional aromatherapy massage using soothing oils such as lavender is also very beneficial for reducing stress and inducing sleep – often before the session is finished!
- Other measures: yoga and meditation; chamomile or lavender herbal tea. For more stubborn cases of insomnia, valarian oil can be used in place of lavender...but do not use it for more than 2 weeks at a stretch, due to its potency.

## JETLAG
The symptoms of jetlag after a long flight are well

recognized: sleep disturbances, disorientation, nervous fatigue and dehydration. Due to its regulating effect on the systems of the body, lavender can be a great aid in overcoming jet lag problems.

- Freshen up frequently during the flight using a little lavender water, or inhale lavender oil from a tissue. In addition, use a lavender moisturizing cream to prevent dryness of the skin.
- After arriving, if possible, take a long bath using 8–10 drops of lavender – this helps readjust the physiological and psychological rhythms.
- To help revive body and mind, use a stimulating oil such as rosemary (5–10 drops) in the bath.

*See also* **Fatigue**

## LABOUR
– *see* **Pregnancy and Childbirth**

## LARYNGITIS
Laryngitis is characterized by a sore throat, hoarseness or a temporary loss of voice brought on by an infection such as bronchitis or flu, or due to over-straining the vocal chords.

- Add 5–10 drops of lavender to a glass of warm water, mix well and gargle. Repeat at least 2 or 3 times a day.
- For a dry cough, make up a concentrated chest rub by mixing 5 drops of lavender with 5 drops of sandalwood in 1 dessertspoon of carrier oil and apply to the chest and throat. Repeat at least twice a day.
- Other oils of benefit: tea tree, eucalyptus and benzoin.

*See also* **Infectious Illnesses**

**LEUCORRHOEA/PRURITIS**
Leucorrhoea is an inflammation of the vagina caused by a proliferation of unwanted bacteria or fungi, which can have a variety of causes. Symptoms often include a thick white or yellow discharge and severe itching of the vaginal area.

Pruritis or itching is an irritating condition which generally accompanies any type of mild vaginal infection.

- As a sitz bath, add 8–10 drops of lavender oil to a bowl or shallow bath of warm water and soak for 5–10 minutes
- Bathe daily, adding 8–10 drops of lavender to the bath water as a general antiseptic measure.
- Make up a 1 per cent lavender ointment –

using a hypo-allergenic bland cream base (see
instructions page 42). Apply to the affected
area as required.

• In addition, avoid tight clothing, nylon
underwear and harsh bubble baths; take garlic
capsules and keep tea, coffee, alcohol and
spices to a minimum. Bergamot, sandalwood
and especially tea tree may also be used to
treat mild vaginal infections in the same
manner as lavender.

*See also* **Cystitis**

## LICE (PEDICULOSIS)

Lice are small blood-sucking insects which cause
the scalp to become itchy and uncomfortable; they
are a common and recurrent problem among
schoolchildren. Most establishments suffer from
periodical outbreaks from time to time since lice
can pass very quickly from one head of hair to the
next irrespective of hair type. The lice also lay tiny
greyish-white eggs (nits) which attach themselves
firmly to the hair, usually near to the scalp.

Both lice and eggs are quite hard to see and can
be difficult to remove. Lavender oil kills lice, but
not their eggs, so it must be used regularly until
all the eggs have either hatched or been removed.
Although the lavender remedy requires more
persistence than commercial chemical treatments,

it actually improves the quality of the hair rather
than damaging it.

- At the start of an outbreak use a 2–3 per cent
  lavender oil shampoo on a daily basis to prevent
  contamination (see instructions page 42).
- Another tip for lice prevention is eating a
  garlic pearl once a day.
- If lice or eggs are found on the hair, make up
  an alcohol-based scalp rub by adding 5 ml of
  lavender to 25 ml of vodka mixed with 75 ml
  water – leave on for at least an hour
  (overnight if possible), then wash out. Finally,
  comb the hair carefully with a fine-toothed
  comb. Use this preparation at the start of an
  infestation and repeat every 3 days until the
  condition has cleared up. Two or three
  applications will usually do the trick! (Replace
  the alcohol/water base with a vegetable oil
  base if the skin becomes irritated).
- Between treatments, wash the hair daily (if
  possible) with a 2–3 per cent lavender
  shampoo – leave on for 10 minutes before
  washing out. In addition add a little lavender
  oil to the conditioner or final rinse water.
- To prevent reinfection, wash all combs and
  brushes in water to which a few drops of
  lavender oil have been added.
- Other measures: tea tree oil is also effective

against lice when used in the same way as you
would lavender.

## MENOPAUSE

Known as the 'change of life', this is the time
when menstruation ceases. It is frequently
characterized by emotional and physical symptoms
of ill-health such as headaches, hot flushes, depression, rapid mood swings, irritability and the
tendency to put on weight.

Due to its regulating and balancing effect,
lavender is particularly valuable in helping the
body to adjust at this difficult time.

• Use lavender oil in baths, vaporizers and for
  massage, according to specific symptoms.

*See also* **Anxiety, Depression, Headaches,
Mood Swings/Hysteria, Stress**

## MIGRAINE

Migraine is most commonly a food-related
complaint, but an attack can also be triggered by
an increase in stress or anxiety. Although aromatherapy is best used as a preventative measure by
promoting relaxation as a part of one's everyday
lifestyle, lavender can also ease the pain and
severity of an attack.

- Apply a cold compress to the temples, using a few drops of lavender oil.
- As a preventative measure, use lavender (or other soothing oils) on a daily basis in baths, vaporizers, for massage or as perfume.

## MOOD SWINGS/HYSTERIA

Hysteria is a term which is no longer used in modern medical practice, not least because it is a condition which is very difficult to define. It has, however, survived as the adjective 'hysterical', usually applied pejoratively to women to describe a certain type of uncontrolled or unpredictable behaviour of a demonstrative emotional character. In spite of its negative associations it is a real and definable condition.

Mood swings, like hysteria, are often associated only with women – especially as a premenstrual or menopausal symptom. They are also, however, a common side-effect of stress. Swings in mood tend to range from hyperactivity and elation on the one hand, to physical exhaustion and depression on the other.

Lavender oil has long been prescribed for hysterical outbursts, a lack of emotional stability, and mood swings:

*Because of its primarily balancing nature, it is of great value in helping people who are in an unbalanced*

*emotional state — hysteria, manic depression or widely*
*fluctuating moods.*[20]

*For treatment, see* **Stress**

## MUSCULAR ACHES AND PAINS

Muscular aches and pains are a common afflic-
tion caused either by physical over-exertion or
by psychological stress and strain. Many people,
for example, carry tension in their necks and
shoulders which over a period of time causes the
muscles to become tight and painful.

> *I was troubled by acute pain and spasm in my neck*
> *muscles...I massaged lavender into my neck which*
> *greatly reduced the pain and muscle spasm. I also felt*
> *soothed by the odour and this was useful as my pain*
> *often made me quite distressed.*[21]

* Soaking in a hot bath is an easy and effective
  way of relaxing the muscles and bringing
  instant pain relief...8–10 drops of lavender oil
  added to the water will increase the benefits
  further due to its analgesic (pain-killing) and
  penetrative qualities.
* Muscular aches and pains respond well to local
  massage — add about 9 drops of lavender to 1
  tbsp of carrier oil and rub into the affected area.
* To relieve muscular spasm or cramp — or if a
  particular area is very tight — massage with neat
  lavender oil or apply a hot compress to which a

few drops of lavender oil have been added.

- A few drops of lavender rubbed into the muscles before and immediately after strenuous sport can help prevent muscular aches and pains from developing.
- Other oils of benefit: tea tree, marjoram, rosemary, black pepper and chamomile (best used in combination with lavender).

## NAUSEA

Feelings of nausea can arise from a variety of different causes including motion or travel sickness, a viral infection, digestive problems, pregnancy or emotional anxiety or tension. Lavender is indicated specifically for sickness due to 'nerves' or an emotional upset, especially if the upset is accompanied by digestive symptoms.

- Inhale lavender directly from a tissue, or vaporize in the room.
- For nausea with indigestion, gently massage the solar plexus/abdomen in a clockwise direction using 3 drops of lavender in 1 tsp carrier oil.
- Other oils: chamomile may be used in a similar way to lavender; peppermint is indicated for travel sickness.

*See also* **Shock**

**NERVOUS TENSION**
– *see* **Stress**

**PALPITATIONS (TACHYCARDIA)**
This is a general term used to describe an irregular heartbeat, either 'missing a beat' or a rapid 'fluttering' of the heart. It can be brought on by exercise but is usually associated with high blood-pressure or stress; it is especially common during the menopause.

• Inhalations of lavender can help calm a rapidly beating heart, although ylang ylang is recognized as the most useful oil for palpitations.
• Regular aromatic bathing and massage using ylang ylang, lavender, neroli, rose or chamomile also help to reduce stress levels and anxiety (which often trigger tachycardia).

*See also* **High Blood-pressure, Menopause, Stress**

**PERIODS (PAINFUL)**
Caused by uterine spasm during menstruation, the frequency and severity of period pains are often also associated with diet and underlying emotional factors.

The soothing effect of lavender, combined with

its excellent analgesic and antispasmodic properties, makes it an excellent remedy for period pains.

- Gently massage the abdomen and lower back with 6 drops of lavender in 2 tsps carrier oil.
- Hot compresses (or a hot water bottle) to which a few drops of lavender have been added placed on the abdomen can help relieve pain.
- Relaxing in a hot lavender bath eases pain and also soothes away stress and tension.
- Other oils of benefit: chamomile, clary sage and marjoram (best used in combination with lavender).

## PERFUME USES

Lavender can be used neat as a perfume to be dabbed on the wrist or behind the ears. It can also be used to perfume linen, paper, leather, pot-pourris or any other object — applied neat, it does not leave a greasy mark. However, the most traditional way of using lavender as a perfume is in the form of an eau-de-cologne, or blended toilet-water. 'Lavender water' was originally prepared by distilling freshly picked lavender flowers which had previously been immersed for a few days in alcohol. Modern lavender water, by contrast, is made by diluting the essential oil with alcohol and then blending it with other ingredients. This is different from the simple 'lavender water' which is produced as a by-product of the distillation process. A simple lavender water can be made as follows:

570 ml/1 pint fairly weak alcohol
125 ml/4 fl oz distilled water
10 drops lavender oil
5 drops rose oil
3 drops ylang ylang oil (in place of the traditional musk)
Mix well and keep in a sealed container for 2–3 weeks before using.

## PERSPIRATION (EXCESSIVE)

Lavender can be used as an excellent disinfectant and deodorant – with a fresh, pleasing scent.

* Add 5–10 drops of lavender to a bowl of warm water and soak the feet nightly for 5 minutes.
* As a quick measure, a few drops of lavender oil can be rubbed into the soles of the feet or beneath the arms in the morning. (Tea tree oil can also be used as a deodorant in the same fashion.)

## PETS/ANIMAL CARE

Essential oils are increasingly employed for the

treatment of common ailments in veterinary practice and for the care of domestic pets –
particularly dogs, cats and horses.

• Fleas – use lavender shampoo (see instructions
  page 42) on a daily basis – leave for 3–5
  minutes before washing out. Afterwards or
  between washes wipe the coat with a moist
  sponge sprinkled with 10–20 drops of pure oil.
  This also improves the condition of the coat.
• Lice – sprinkle the coat with 10–20 drops of
  lavender oil and brush through. Repeat daily.
• Rashes – apply pure lavender oil or, if needed
  to treat a larger area, use lavender diluted to
  2.5 per cent with a light carrier oil or cream
  (see instructions page 42).
• Cuts/itches/scabs/insect bites/bumps – apply
  pure lavender oil. Repeat 2–3 times a day
  until healed.
• Other measures: tea tree oil may be used in a
  similar fashion.

## PREGNANCY AND CHILDBIRTH

Using essential oils during pregnancy and to help
with childbirth can be very beneficial in a variety
of ways, because they operate on both a
physiological and a psychological level.

Lavender is *the* most useful oil during pregnancy, not only because it is very safe but also

because of its predominantly calming/healing/balancing character.

> Relaxation and rest are the two very important factors during pregnancy in order that the mother and child enjoy their togetherness. Lavender oil is very useful for this purpose. It is a lovely all-rounder...[22]

Because of the sensitivity of the growing child, however, all essential oils (including lavender) should only be used at half the usual amount during pregnancy.

- An excellent oil to help prevent stretch marks can be made by blending 3 drops of lavender with 1 tbs wheatgerm oil – for light massage daily to the belly and breasts. This oil can also help to get rid of existing stretch marks. Wheatgerm oil can also be rubbed into the perineum to help prepare for the birth.
- Aromatic bathing is a great pleasure and relief, especially towards the end of pregnancy. Add 3–5 drops of lavender to the bath, and relax in the aromatic vapours.
- Gentle massage using lavender (in dilution) can be very enjoyable during pregnancy and can help with a wide variety of problems such as back pain, anxiety or fatigue.
- Haemorrhoids are common during pregnancy. To relieve itching, massage the affected area

with an oily cream or a soapy solution to which a few drops each of lavender, bergamot and geranium have been added.

- Pain relief during labour can be aided by firm massage to the lower back using the following blend: 3 drops each of lavender and clary sage in 1 tbs carrier oil.

- During the birth, and in preparing to bring the baby into the home, the use of vaporized oils to scent the environment can be very conducive to creating an uplifting, relaxed mood. They also prevent the spread of airborne bacteria. Lavender has been used since Roman times to help facilitate childbirth and is the most traditional oil to vaporize in the room during labour.

- To help heal the perineum after the birth, add 5 drops of lavender to a shallow bath, and soak. Repeat each day.[23]

- Postnatal depression can be helped by the use of lavender in burners, baths and for massage.

*Note:* Some essential oils should be avoided altogether during pregnancy, including basil, clove, cinnamon leaf, hyssop, juniper, marjoram, myrrh, sage and thyme. The following oils are also best avoided during the first four months of pregnancy: fennel, peppermint and rosemary.

## PREMENSTRUAL TENSION

The symptoms of PMT are various: on a physical level these may include fluid retention, tender breasts, headaches, nausea or a swollen abdomen; while on an emotional level symptoms commonly include depression, sudden mood swings, weepiness or unpredictable behaviour. Considering the overall 'harmonizing' or 'balancing' effect of lavender on the whole system, it is a very useful aid for women who suffer from PMT, both physically and emotionally.

> *A married woman aged 26 found that she could no longer put up with her terrible PMT. Her moods were awfully black, she was very irritable, suffered from cramps in her abdomen and lower back, and of vomiting...I blended the following oils for her: chamomile, lavender, geranium and melissa (to be used in the bath and in a massage oil for two weeks before her period)...she has now had four periods and says that both mentally and physically it has a been a huge success.*[24]

- Use lavender in baths and in a vaporizer during the 10 days prior to menstruation, and throughout the duration of the period.
- A regular massage treatment with lavender can be very helpful. For self-treatment, mix 6 drops of lavender oil in 1 tbsp light carrier

oil such as grapeseed, and apply gently to the abdomen and lower back.

- A nutritional approach to PMT has been developed over the past few years with excellent results. Supplements of Evening Primrose Oil, vitamin B$_6$ and the B complex have also proved invaluable.
- Other oils of benefit: rose, geranium, chamomile, neroli and clary sage.

## PRURITIS (ITCHING)
– *see* **Leucorrhoea/Pruritis**

## RHEUMATISM
The term 'rheumatism' is used medically to describe a whole range of disorders which involve pain in the muscles or joints, including the various forms of arthritis and gout. Generally speaking, however, rheumatism refers specifically to muscular pain, whereas arthritis and gout are associated with pain located within the joints themselves.

Lavender can help to ease rheumatic pain due to its analgesic qualities – it also increases local blood circulation and enhances mobility. Since rheumatism, like arthritis, is aggravated by an accumulation of toxins in the system, diet and lifestyle should also be assessed (by, for example, a qualified nutritionist/herbalist/aromatherapist).

- Massage is itself very helpful for rheumatic pains because it stimulates the circulation and helps remove toxins. Make up a concentrated massage oil by mixing 30 drops of lavender oil with 50 ml of a vegetable carrier oil. Apply twice daily.
- Add 8–10 drops of lavender oil to the bath water for pain relief.
- Other oils of benefit include chamomile, tea tree, marjoram and rosemary (best used in combination).

*See also* **Arthritis, Muscular Aches and Pains**

**SCABIES**
Scabies is a highly contagious skin disease caused by the itch mite *sarcoptes scabiei*. Scabies is common in sheepfarming areas, where it is commonly transmitted from the wool of the sheep to the farm workers. It can also be picked up in changing rooms, and even from handling coins – it does not require close contact to pass from one person to another. The female mites lay their eggs under the skin, and as the newly hatched mites burrow their way out this causes severe irritation and itching – especially at night. Small red pimples may appear and scratching can lead to sores which can then become infected. Common areas to be affected are the groin, penis, nipples and the skin between the fingers.

- Wash the skin gently, then treat the affected area with a 5 per cent lavender non-oily cream or gel (see instructions page 42) – repeat 2 or 3 times a day.
- As a matter of routine, add 8–10 drops of lavender to the bath water as a disinfectant measure.
- During treatment, scrupulous attention to hygiene is essential. To prevent re-infection, change and wash all pillowcases, towels, bedding, clothes (especially woollens), etc. using a few drops of lavender oil in the washing water – sponge the mattress down using a 10 per cent solution in alcohol.
- Other oils of benefit: tea tree, peppermint.

## SHINGLES (ZONA)
– *see* **Chickenpox**

## SHOCK/VERTIGO
Lavender water was at one time used as a remedy for vertigo, 'swoonings' or 'faintings' brought on by shock. Dr Valnet recommends lavender as an evening bath oil for 'weak and delicate children' and for 'shock, tantrums, etc.'. It also helps allay the effects of clinical shock or of stopping a severe addiction and, as a regulating agent and anti-depressant, it helps overcome the psychological shock of injury:

> *Lavender is both a habit-breaker and a crisis-smoother.*[25]

- Inhale neat lavender oil from a tissue, or add 8–10 drops to the bath to help cope with the emotional after-effects of a shock.
- Other measures: take the Bach Flower Remedy 'Rescue Remedy' immediately.

## SKIN CARE

Lavender is one of the most useful skin care oils because although it has excellent antiseptic properties it is very mild to the skin. It has been used as an ingredient in cosmetics for centuries and its effects have been well tried and tested. It is suited to all types of complexion, particularly oily and mature (wrinkled) skin.

Lavender is also an excellent cicatrizant or wound-healing oil which promotes tissue or cell regeneration and prevents scarring. It is these combined properties that make lavender a valuable oil for all types of injury to the skin and also for the treatment of a wide range of specific skin conditions.

- As a cleanser/toner for everyday skin care (especially for dry or mature skin), blend 15 drops each of rose and lavender essential oils with 25 ml of witchhazel and 75 ml distilled

water (or another flower water) and apply
morning and night before moisturizing the skin.
- For moisturizing the skin, blend 3 drops of
lavender with 1 tsp wheatgerm oil (or a
moisturizing cream); apply twice daily.
- For a reviving cosmetic vinegar to strengthen
the acid mantle of the skin, mix 6 parts
rosewater, 1 part spirit of lavender and 2 parts
vinegar.
- There are many other essential oils that are
particularly beneficial for the skin, including
tea tree (for oily skin), rose (for dry/mature
skin) and geranium (for combination skin).

*See also* **Acne, Cracked Skin, Dermatitis/
Eczema**

**SPLINTERS, INFECTED**
After removing a splinter, always apply a drop of
lavender oil to prevent infection. Splinters can be
dangerous if they do become infected – often
because a small portion of the splinter remains
embedded in the skin.

- If the splinter is infected, sore and with pus:
clean the area gently, apply pure lavender oil,
then cover with a clay poultice or plaster
(adhesive bandage) and leave for 2 hours to
help draw it out. Remove the splinter with a

pair of tweezers – repeat the procedure if this
does not work – then apply a few drops of
lavender and cover with a plaster (adhesive
bandage).
• Other oils of benefit: tea tree, chamomile (for
  inflammation).

## SPOTS
– *see* **Acne**

## SPRAINS
As an analgesic and anti-inflammatory agent,
lavender is useful for treating sprains.

• Prepare a cold compress to which a few drops
  of lavender (or chamomile) have been added,
  apply to the injury. Repeat as often as possible
  to reduce the swelling. Do *not* massage the
  injured area; wrap it in a bandage and rest as
  much as possible.

## STRESS
'Stress' is not an illness as such but a 'multi-
dimensional syndrome' which can cause a wide
range of physical ailments and psychological
problems ranging from high blood-pressure,
headaches or digestive complaints to feelings of
constant tiredness, depression or nervous anxiety.
Stress also weakens the immune system and, in the

long term, makes an individual more susceptible to all kinds of disease.

Recent research indicates that stress is most probably a causative factor or a trigger for many of the so-called 'civilization' diseases such as cancer, ME, stroke, and AIDS. Material proof of the widespread sense of 'dis-ease' experienced today is shown by the high consumption of tranquillizers and stimulants, although it is well known that addiction, toxicosis and other side-effects can be caused by these drugs if they are taken regularly.

Any treatment which can help to de-stress or revitalize the organism without producing detrimental side-effects is, therefore, of great value.

> *The possibility of applying new therapies to these widespread psycho-neurosis is therefore of considerable importance...essential oils that are employed in aromatherapy, in the appropriate doses, are harmless to the organism and do not cause troubles like those produced by the ordinary psychological drugs. Very conclusive experiments in this direction have been carried out in various clinics for nervous diseases, on patients affected by hysteria or psychic depression.*[26]

Stress-related problems are an area in which aromatherapy enjoys a great deal of success, due to the powerful combination of touch and smell. During a massage, the essential oils themselves also interact with and de-stress the body in two ways: through inhalation (primarily psychological effects) and through dermal absorption (primarily physiological effects). By easing the problem at its source, rather than by treating the individual symptoms, aromatherapy is especially valuable for those who suffer from a number of different responses to stress simultaneously. In the words of Dr Ann Coxon:

> For instance, a person who has a difficult ongoing life situation, who has high blood-pressure which needs one set of tablets, indigestion requiring another set of tablets, back pain that would actually be contra-indicated in view of the indigestion, and so on. One could go on with that patient forever. And they invariably end up with 15 pots of tablets, total confusion and a sense of dependency on the doctors. Obviously, the approach of holistic treatment is to help enable people to manage their primary life situation, and the ability of aromatherapy to get at the knot, at the stress reaction itself within the body without using yet more pharmacological treatment is terribly important.[27]

Lavender is possibly the most useful oil employed in this context because of its regulating effect on the nervous functions and its versatile nature. Indeed, lavender is indicated for all the symptoms mentioned above, for it reduces blood-pressure (especially in combination with massage), eases back pain, soothes indigestion and reduces any emotional anxiety. It is in such cases that lavender really comes into its own!

* Use lavender in baths, vaporizers, massage, perfumes, etc. for its de-stressing effects.

*For specific symptoms, see* **Anxiety**, **Depression**, **Fatigue**, **High Blood-pressure**, **Insomnia**, **Mood Swings/Hysteria**, **Palpitations**

**SUNBURN**
Due to its excellent healing and analgesic properties, lavender can provide instant relief from heat rash or red and sore skin – it can also prevent blistering.

* For large areas, make a lotion using 12 drops of lavender oil in 1 tbsp of distilled water (or a water-based gel to which 5–10 per cent lavender oil has been added) and dab the area gently.
* For severe patches of sunburn apply lavender oil neat.
* Other measures: soaking in a lukewarm bath containing 6–8 drops of lavender or chamomile roman is very soothing; tea tree is also a very effective sunburn remedy when used in the same manner as lavender.

*See also* **Burns**

**ULCERS (VARICOSE AND TROPICAL)**
Varicose ulcers can form on the lower legs when
the veins are not functioning properly, often as
a result of varicose veins. Elderly people are
particularly prone to this condition, especially if
they suffer from poor circulation – some merely
have to scratch the skin on their lower legs to
develop a sore which can be very slow to heal.

> *Patient with a long-standing varicose ulcer. All else had
> failed. [Treated with lavender.] Healed in 17 days.*[28]

Tropical ulcers (also known as 'naga sores') usually
occur in hot, humid climates. Again a large
painless sore develops, often on the feet or legs,
due to a bacterial infection, poor nutrition or
environmental factors.

Gattefossé and Valnet used lavender successfully
for the treatment of ulcers (see page 19).

> *Infected ulcerated lesion of the lower third of the left
> leg. 24th December first application of lavender. 31st
> December: improvement, the purulent suppurating base
> was granulating and pink. By 16th January, the sore
> was half its original size. By 10th February, it had
> healed completely.*[29]

- As a preventative measure, apply a 5 per cent
  lavender cream/oil (see instructions page 42)

    to the lower legs on a daily basis.

- To treat an ulcer, bathe the sore gently with a warm diluted solution of lavender oil (by adding a few drops to a bowl of distilled/boiled water). Then apply a 10 per cent lavender cream (see instructions page 42), or cover with a pad which has been saturated in a solution of 3 parts olive oil to 1 part lavender oil.
- Tea tree oil may be used in the same manner (or in combination with lavender).

## VAGINAL INFECTIONS
– *see* **Leucorrhoea/Pruritis**

## WHOOPING COUGH
Whooping cough, which is characterized by a sudden intake of breath or 'whoop' after a bout of coughing, can develop after a respiratory infection such as a cold, and usually affects children under the age of eight.

    Lavender's antispasmodic properties have a calming effect and help combat the primary infection.

- Use lavender in vaporizers in the bedroom, for the course of the illness, and in steaming hot inhalations (to soothe the bouts of coughing).
- Apply a hot compress to the chest using a few

drops of lavender to facilitate breathing, or
massage neat into the throat.

## ZONA (SHINGLES)
– *see* **Chickenpox**

# The Different Types of Lavender Oil

There has long been some confusion over the correct botanical name for 'true' lavender, but the exact derivation for the commercially grown plant today is *L. angustifolia* Mill. subsp. *angustifolia*[1]. Apart from 'true' lavender there are principally three other types which are widespread throughout Europe and the Mediterranean region and are used for producing essential oils: spike lavender (*L. latifolia*), lavandin (*L.* x *intermedia*) and stoechas lavender (*L. stoechas*).

SPIKE LAVENDER, also known as Aspic, Lesser Lavender, *Nardus italica* or Broad-leaved Lavender (*L. latifolia, L. spica*)
An evergreen sub-shrub up to 1 m (3½ ft) high, with lance-shaped leaves and dull greyish-blue flowers. It is found all along the Mediterranean coast, growing at altitudes of up to 800 m (2,624 ft) and cultivated on the south coast of France, in

Italy, but most of all in Spain. The Spanish and French varieties represent two different chemotypes: the former is high in ketones, notably camphor (up to 60 per cent), making it a good mucolytic, stimulating and very penetrating oil but also quite toxic (contra-indicated for epilepsy); the latter is lower in ketones but contains more cineole and linalol, which makes it a useful expectorant. Spike lavender is current in the *British Herbal Pharmacopoeia*, where it is indicated for flatulent dyspepsia, colic, depressive headache, and the oil (topically) for rheumatic pain. The French oil has a more delicate scent, but both it and the Spanish variety have a harsher fragrance than true lavender.

LAVANDIN or 'Bastard Lavender' (*L. x intermedia, L. hybrida, L. hortensis, L. burnatii*)
Lavandin is a cross between true lavender (*L. angustifolia*) and spike lavender (*L. latifolia*), and due to its hybrid nature can take a variety of forms. In general it is a larger plant than *L. angustifolia*, though its flowers may be violet-blue like true lavender or greyish like spike. If the resultant cross is closer to true lavender it is called lavender 'abrial'; if closer to spike lavender it is called lavender 'reydovan'.

Lavender 'abrial' contains up to 30 per cent esters (mainly linalyl acetate) and is a good anti-infectious oil and quite sedative in effect. Sixty years ago lavandin only occurred in its wild form, but now it is commonly cultivated due to its hardy nature and because it yields more essential oil than either true lavender or spike. Its scent, however, is less refined than that of true lavender; nor can the oil be used as a substitute medicinally. (A concrete and absolute are also produced by solvent extraction).

LAVENDER STOECHAS, 'French' Lavender, Stickadore, Stichados, Cassidony or Arabian stoechas (*L. stoechas*)

A smaller shrub than true lavender, with dark purple, compact flowers. It grows in Italy, France, Spain and North Africa, although it is not as extensively cultivated as the three former varieties. The oil has a camphorous odour, more like rosemary than lavender, which is used in perfumes and soap, and contains a high proportion of the ketones camphor and fenchone, which makes it considerably toxic. It is nevertheless useful when used in dilution for chronic sinusitis, bronchitis and upper respiratory infections. Six sub-species exist.

OTHER SUB-SPECIES There are several sub-species of lavender (*L. angustifolia*), the two principal sub-species being *L. delphinensis* and *L. fragrans*. Different sub-species or chemotypes have also evolved according to the soil, altitude and habitat, for example six varieties have been developed in Bulgaria alone through a selection programme, including 'Kazanluc', 'Karlovo', 'Hemus', 'Aroma', 'Svezhest' and 'Venets'. In addition, true lavender and spike lavender cross-hybridize with ease, and over the centuries have interbred in the wild, as well as in cultivation, to produce a wide variety of plants. The resulting cultivars, which may be first generation or subsequent generation plants, have been given different names according to their origination, such as 'Hidcote Pink', 'Bowles Early' or 'Dwarf Blue'. There are also many cultivars of lavandin and spike lavender.

Around 50 different species can be seen in the UK at the National Lavender Collection, Caley Mill, Norfolk PE31 7JE.

~❦~

# The Constituents of Lavender Oil

dimethyl sulphide (trace)

1,3(E),5(Z),8(Z)-undecatetraene (0.01%)

acetone (0.08%)

sabinene hydrate (0.11%)

pentanal (trace)

trans-linalool oxide-furanoid (0.16%)

methoxyhexane (0.09%)

camphenilone (trace)

tricyclene (0.01%)

camphor (0.45%)

α-pinene (0.34%)

linalool (17.81%)

α-thujene (0.22%)

linalyl acetate (21.84%)

prenol[1a] (trace)

β-bergamotene (0.12%)

camphene (0.22%)

α-santalene (1.11%)

butyl acetate (0.06%)

bornyl acetate (0.55%)

hexanal (trace)

α-bergamotene (0.15%)

β-pinene (0.18%)

sabinene (0.05%)

butyl propionate (0.01%)

butyl isobutyrate (0.02%)

δ-3-carene (0.13%)

myrcene (1.27%)

α-phellandrene (0.07%)

α-terpinene (0.11%)

limonene (0.42%)

1,8-cineole (0.91%)

butyl butyrate (0.25%)

2-hexenal (trace)

(Z)-β-ocimene (8.23%)

γ-terpinene (0.38%)

(E)-β-ocimene (6.24%)

3-octanone (1.39%)

hexyl acetate (0.55%)

p-cymene (0.29%)

terpinolene (0.15%)

octanal (trace)

3-octyl acetate (0.18%)

lavandulyl acetate (7.30%)

terpinen-4-ol (6.43%)

β-caryophyllene (8.00%)

hexyl tiglate (0.10%)

β-santalene (0.02%)

β-farnesene (1.98%)

lavandulol (1.17%)

α-humulene (0.25%)

cryptone (0.18%)

α-terpineol (1.00%)

borneol (1.06%)

germacrene D (0.88%)

neryl acetate (0.53%)

cis-linalool oxide-pyranoid (trace)

geranyl acetate (0.96%)

carvone (trace)

trans-linalool oxide pyranoid (trace)

γ-cadinene (0.25%)

tricyclo-ekα-santalal (0.05%)

nerol (0.23%)

cuminaldehyde (0.13%)

hexyl propionate (0.02%)

hexyl isobutyrate (0.08%)

hexanol (0.02%)

ocimene oxide (trace)

3,7-dimethylocta-2,4,
6-triene (0.03%)

1-octen-3-yl acetate
(2.49%)

3-octanol (0.18%)

galbanolene[2b] (0.11%)

nonanal (trace)

rose furan (0.01%)

hexyl butyrate (0.38%)

butyl tiglate (0.11%)

1-octen-3-ol (0.48%)

cis-linalool oxide-furanoid (0.16%)

epoxy-linalyl acetate
(0.02%)

geraniol (0.43%)

p-cymen-8-ol (0.17%)

epoxy-$\alpha$-santalene
(trace)

hotrienol (trace)

linalyl hexanoate
(0.11%)

butyl benzoate (trace)

$\beta$-caryophyllene oxide
(trace)

$\alpha$-photosantalol A
(0.10%)

isocaryophyllene oxide
(0.33%)

cubenol (trace)

T-cadinol (0.31%)

thymol (trace)

FROM PERFUMER & FLAVORIST 18 (JAN./FEB. 1993)

[a] prenol is also known as 2-methyl-but-2-en-4-ol

[b] galbanolene is also known as 1,3(E),5(Z)-
undecatriene

# References

## Introduction

1. Extract from 'L'histoire de la Jouvencelle, Lieutenante des Oiseaux', a story from *Mille et une Nuits* (A Thousand and One Nights) cited in C. Meunier, *Lavandes et Lavandins* (Paris: Edisud, 1985), p. 5 transl. by S. Alcock.
2. C. Isherwood, *A Bunch of Sweet Lavender* (Hitchin, Paternoster and Hales, brochure on the lavender industry [copy in Miss Lewis' private lavender museum in 1977]).

## Chapter 1

1. S. Festing, *The Story of Lavender* (London Borough of Sutton Libraries and Arts Services, 1982), p. 31.
2. *Mitcham News*, 20th July 1934
3. From a poem by M. E. Davies in *Hitchin Grammar School Magazine* c.1960, cited in Festing, *Story of Lavender*, p. 39.
4. A. K. Singh, S. Ashok and O. P. Virmani, 'Cultivation of Lavender for its Oil – A Review', *Current Research on Medicinal and Aromatic Plants* 5.1 (1983), p. 54.

## Chapter 2

1. Dioscorides, *The Greek Herbal* (ed. R. T. Gunther; Oxford: Oxford University Press, 1937).
2. Y. R. Naves and B. Mazuyer, *Natural Perfume Materials* (New York: Reinhold, 1947), p.5.
3. Hildegarde, *Patrologia Latina* (ed. Migne; vol. 197, from *Liber subtilitatum diversarum naturarum creaturarum*, 1150–60).
4. J. Gerarde, cited in R. Tisserand, *The Art of Aromatherapy* (C. W. Daniel, 1979), p. 246.
5. N. Culpeper, *Culpeper's Complete Herbal* (W. Foulsham & Co. Ltd, 1952), p. 210.

6. W. Salmon, cited in Festing, *Story of Lavender*, p. 28.

*Chapter 3*

1. M. Grieve, *A Modern Herbal* (Penguin, 1982), p. 472.
2. Dr J. Valnet, *The Practice of Aromatherapy* (C. W. Daniel, 1980), p. 148.
3. R. M. Gattefossé, *Gattefossé's Aromatherapy* (C. W. Daniel, 1993), p. 106.
4. M. Maury, *Marguerite Maury's Guide to Aromatherapy* (C. W. Daniel, 1989), p. 85.
5. 'Aromatherapy on the Wards', *International Journal of Aromatherapy* 1.2 (1988), p. 8.
6. J. Guillemain, A. Rousseau and P. Delaveau, in *Ann. Pharm. Fr* 47.6 (1989), pp. 337–43.
7. A. Y. Leung, *Encyclopedia of Common Natural Ingredients* (New York: Wiley, 1980), p. 215.
8. M. Hardy, 'Sweet Scented Dreams', *International Journal of Aromatherapy* 3.2 (1991), p. 13.
9. G. Buchbauer, L. Jirovetz, W. Jager, H. Dietrich and C. Plank, in *Z. Naturforsch C* 46 (Nov.–Dec. 1991), pp. 1067–72.
10. R. Lewis, *Natural Therapies Database*, Aromatherapy Vol. I, printed by R. Harris, p. 13.
11. A. Woolfson and D. Hewitt, 'Intensive Aromacare', *International Journal of Aromatherapy* 4.2 (1992), p. 13.
12. J. Buckle, 'Aromatherapy – Research in Practice', *Nursing Times* 89.20 (May 19, 1993), p. 32.
13. Buckle, 'Aromatherapy', p. 35.

*Chapter 4*

1. A. O. Tucker and B. M. Lawrence, 'Herbs, Spices and Medicinal Plants', vol. 2 (Oryx Press, 1987).
2. Cited in Festing, *Story of Lavender*, p. 77.

*Chapter 5*

1. J. Lawless, *Aromatherapy and the Mind* (Thorsons, 1994), p. 77.
2. Cited in Tisserand, *Art of Aromatherapy*, p. 100.
3. P. Holmes, 'Lavender Oil – A Study in Contradictions', *International Journal of Aromatherapy* 4.2, 1992.

*A–Z*

1. A. Marshall, 'Problem Skin', *Aromatherapy Quarterly* 8 (1985), p. 12.
2. Lawless, *Aromatherapy and the Mind*, p. 77.
3. Lawless, *Aromatherapy and the Mind*, p. 80.
4. S. Macnish, 'The Soothing Touch', *International Journal of Aromatherapy* 3.2 (1991), p. 19.

5. D. Falt, 'Asthma', *International Journal of Aromatherapy* 3.4 (1991), p. 32.
6. Gattefossé, 'Dr Marchand's Observations', in *idem*, *Gattefossé's Aromatherapy*, p. 90.
7. M. Dambach-Sinclair, 'Miraculous Healing', *International Journal of Aromatherapy* 3.4 (1991), p. 32.
8. Gattefossé, 'Dr Marchand's Observations', in *idem*, *Gattefossé's Aromatherapy*, p. 90.
9. Dr Ann Coxon, Consultant Physician and Neurologist, from 'Prescribing Aromatherapy', *Aromatherapy Quarterly* 31 (Winter 1991), p. 9.
10. Grieve, *Modern Herbal*, p. 472.
11. Dr T. Betts, 'Sniffing the Breeze', *Aromatherapy Quarterly* 40 (1994), p. 22.
12. Meunier, *Lavandes*, p. 198.
13. P. Allardice, *Lavender* (Robert Hale, 1991), p. 57.
14. 'Progress in Essential Oils: Lavender Oil', *Perfumer & Flavorist* 18 (Jan./Feb. 1993), p. 58.
15. P. Davis, *Aromatherapy – an A–Z* (C. W. Daniel, 1988), p. 166.
16. Davis, *A–Z*, p. 173.
17. Holmes, 'Study in Contradictions', p. 22.
18. Valnet, *Practice of Aromatherapy*, p. 148.
19. A. Ascham, *The Little Herball* (1525).
20. Davis, *A–Z*, p. 200.
21. C. Cunningham, 'Whiplash', *International Journal of Aromatherapy* 3.1 (1991), p. 24.
22. J. Basnyet, from a lecture given to midwives entitled 'Aromatherapy in Ante- and Postnatal Care', *Aromatherapy Times* 18 (Winter 1992), p. 11
23. A. Dale, *Journal of Advanced Nursing* (1994) issue 19, pp. 89–96.
24. J. Gingell, 'PMT', *Aromatherapy Quarterly* 8 (1985), p. 12.
25. Holmes, 'Study in Contradictions', p. 21.
26. Rovesti, cited in Tisserand, *Art of Aromatherapy*, p. 98.
27. Coxon, 'Prescribing Aromatherapy', p. 9.
28. Gattefossé, 'Dr Meurisse's Observations', in *idem*, *Gattefossé's Aromatherapy*, p. 94.
29. Gattefossé, 'Dr Marchand's Observations', in *idem*, *Gattefossé's Aromatherapy*, p. 90.

## Appendix A

1. A. O. Tucker and K. J. W. Hensen, 'The Cultivars of Lavender and Lavandin', *Baileya* 22 (1985).

## Appendix B

1. Dr Brian M. Lawrence, 'Progress in Essential Oils' in *Perfumer & Flavorist* (1993) issue no. 18, pp. 58–61.

# Bibliography

P. Allardice, *Lavender* (Robert Hale, 1991).

'Aromatherapy on the Wards', *International Journal of Aromatherapy* 1.2 (1988).

Aqua Oleum, *The Essential Oil Catalogue* (Aqua Oleum, 1994).

J. Basnyet, 'Aromatherapy in Ante- and Postnatal Care', *Aromatherapy Times* 18 (Winter 1992).

Dr T. Betts, 'Sniffing the Breeze', *Aromatherapy Quarterly* 40 (1994).

R. Blackwell, 'An insight into Aromatic Oils: Lavender and Tea Tree', *British Journal of Phytotherapy* 2.1 (Spring 1991).

*British Herbal Pharmacopeia* (BHMA, 1983).

J. and M. Brunner, 'Lavender and Marjoram', *The Herbal Review* (Winter 1982).

G. Buchbauer, L. Jirovetz, W. Jager, H. Dietrich and C. Plank, in *Z. Naturforsch C* 46 (Nov.–Dec. 1991).

J. Buckle, 'Aromatherapy – Research in Practice', *Nursing Times* 89.20 (May 19, 1993).

Dr A. Coxon, 'Prescribing Aromatherapy', *Aromatherapy Quarterly* 31 (Winter 1991).

N. Culpeper, *Culpeper's Complete Herbal* (W. Foulsham & Co. Ltd, 1952).

C. Cunningham, 'Whiplash', *International Journal of Aromatherapy* 3.1 (1991).

M. Dambach-Sinclair, 'Miraculous Healing', *International Journal of Aromatherapy* 3.4 (1991).

P. Davis, *Aromatherapy – an A–Z* (C. W. Daniel, 1988).

Dioscorides, *The Greek Herbal* (ed. R. T. Gunther; Oxford: Oxford University Press, 1937).

Essential Oils Sub-Committee, 'Application of Gas–Liquid Chromatography to the Analysis of Essential Oils. Part 5 – Lavender and Lavandin', *Analyst* 102 (August, 1977), pp. 607–612.

D. Falt, 'Asthma', *International Journal of Aromatherapy* 3.4 (1991).

S. Festing, *The Story of Lavender* (London Borough of Sutton Libraries and Arts Services, 1982).

S. Fischer-Rizzi, *Complete Aromatherapy Handbook* (New York: Sterling, 1990).

R. M. Gattefossé, *Gattefossé's Aromatherapy* (C. W. Daniel, 1993).

J. Gingell, 'PMT', *Aromatherapy Quarterly* 8 (1985).

M. Grieve, *A Modern Herbal* (Penguin, 1982).

N. Groom, *The Perfume Handbook* (Chapman & Hall, 1992).

E. Guenther, *The Essential Oils* (New York: Van Nostrand, 1950).

J. Guillemain, a. Rousseau and P. Delaveau, in *Ann. Pharm. Fr* 47.6 (1989).

M. Hardy, 'Sweet Scented Dreams', *International Journal of Aromatherapy* 3.2 (1991).

Hildegarde, *Patrologia Latina* (ed. Migne; vol. 197, from *Liber subtilitatum diversarum naturarum creaturarum*, 1150–60).

P. Holmes, 'Lavender Oil – A Study in Contradictions', *International Journal of Aromatherapy* 4.2, 1992.

J. Lawless, *the Encyclopaedia of Essential Oils* (Element Books, 1992).

–, *Home Aromatherapy* (Kyle Kathie, 1993).

–, *Aromatherapy and the Mind* (Thorsons, 1994).

A. Y. Leung, *Encyclopedia of Common Natural Ingredients* (New York: Wiley, 1980).

R. Lovell, *A Compleat Herball* (2nd edn, 1665).

S. Macnish, 'The Soothing Touch', *International Journal of Aromatherapy* 3.2 (1991).

M. Maury, *Marguerite Maury's Guide to Aromatherapy* (C. W. Daniel, 1989).

M. Mességué, *Health Secrets of Plants and Herbs* (Pan, 1979).

C. Meunier, *Lavandes et Lavandins* (Paris: Edisud, 1985).

Y. R. Naves and B. Mazuyer, *Natural Perfume Materials* (New York: Reinhold, 1947).

M. Page, *The Observer's Book of Herbs* (F. Warne, 1980).

M. J. Prager and M. A. Miskiewcz, 'Gas Chromatographic-Mass

Spectrometric Analysis, Identification and Detection of Adulteration of Lavender, Lavandin and Spike Lavender Oils', *J. Assoc. Off. Anal. Chem.* 62.6 (1979).

'Progress in Essential Oils: Lavender Oil', *Perfumer & Flavorist* 18 (Jan./Feb. 1993).

B. Salmon, *Nature's Secrets* (Vita Press, 1991).

J. C. Sawyer, 'Lavender: Its Cultivation and Distillation', *The Journal of the Society of Chemical Industry* (May 30th, 1891).

J. Sheen, *Lavender* (Dorling Kindersley, 1991).

A. K. Singh, S. Ashok and O. P. Virmani, 'Cultivation of Lavender for its Oil – A Review', *Current Research on Medicinal and Aromatic Plants* 5.1 (1983).

R. Tisserand, *The Art of Aromatherapy* (C. W. Daniel, 1979).

A. O. Tucker and K. J. W. Hensen, 'The Cultivars of Lavender and Lavandin', *Baileya* 22 (1985).

A. O. Tucker and B. M. Lawrence, 'Herbs, Spices and Medicinal Plants', vol. 2 (Oryx Press, 1987).

Dr J. Valnet, *The Practice of Aromatherapy* (C. W. Daniel, 1980).

A. Woolfson and D. Hewitt, 'Intensive Aromacare', *International Journal of Aromatherapy* 4.2 (1992).

R. C. Wren, *Potter's New Cyclopaedia of Botanical Drugs and Preparations* (C. W. Daniel, 1989).

# Useful Addresses

It is advisable always to buy lavender oil from a reputable supplier, to ensure that it is of the highest quality so as to achieve maximum therapeutic results. Aqua Oleum have many years of experience in the field and provide a wide range of top-quality essential oils including lavender at very competitive prices. They can be purchased from health and wholefood stores, as well as from some chemists, throughout the UK. Mail-order items, carrier oils, burners, individually formulated products and further information can be obtained from:

Aqua Oleum, Unit 3, Lower Wharf, Wallbridge, Stroud, Glos GL5 3JA, UK – Tel: 01453 753555

Aqua Oleum also supply lavender internationally to the following countries:

*Eire*
  Wholefoods Wholesale
  Unit 2D
  Kylemore Industrial
  Estate
  Dublin 10

Soap Opera Ltd
Unit 3 Enterprise Centre
Stafford Street
Nenagh
Co. Tipperary

*US and Canada*
  Natura Trading Ltd
  4454 West 10th Avenue
  Vancouver
  British Columbia
  V6R 2H9

*Japan*
  Raiko Co. Ltd
  4b, 2-2-8 Roppongi
  Minato-Ku
  Tokyo

  Kawahito Trading Office
  Room 308
  Fushu Musashino
  High Raise 3-11-13
  Sakae-cho
  Fushu-shi
  Tokyo 183

*Hong Kong*
  The New Age Shop
  7 Old Bailey Street
  Central

*Taiwan*
  Ecole Internationale
  D'Esthetique D'Europe
  15F 1 547 Kwang Fiu
  South Road
  Hsin Vi Zone
  Taipei

*Norway*
  Terapi Consult AS
  Frysjaveien 27
  0883 Oslo

*Denmark and Sweden*
  Urtekram A/S
  Klostermarken 20
  DK-9550 Mariager
  Denmark

*Finland*
  Luonnonruokatukku
  Aduki Ky
  Kirvesmiehenkatu 10
  00810 Helsinki

For information on Norfolk Lavender Ltd, producers of lavender oil, contact:

Norfolk Lavender Ltd, Caley Mill, Heacham, Norfolk PE31 7JE – Tel: 01485 570384

# Index

abscesses 47–8
absolutes 113
acne 34, 48–9
acupuncture 43
allopathic medicines 43
alopecia 72–3
amounts, for babies and children 58–9
analgesic properties *see* pain relief
animal care 94–5
anti-inflammatory properties 33–4
anti-spasmodic agent 18, 34
anti-toxic properties 18, 38
anti-venomous properties 38
antidote, for poisons 10
antipyretic effects 38
antiseborrhoeic properties 34
antiseptic properties 16, 17, 33–4
anxiety 24–5, 36, 50–51
apoplexy 14
apricot kernel oil 42
'aqua water' 4–5
Arabian stoechas 113
arnica ointment 55
aromatherapy xiv–xvi, 19, 20, 24–5
arthritis 21, 34, 51–2
aspic xvi, 111
asthma 53–4
Atlas cedarwood 82

avocado oil 42

babies 43–4, 58–60
Bach 'Rescue Remedy' 102
bactericidal properties 17, 33–4
balancing properties 35
baldness 72–3
basil 84, 97
bastard lavender *see* lavandin
baths 3, 20–21, 39, 42, 58–9
bee stings 81
benzoin 61, 85
bergamot 49, 51, 64, 65, 67, 70, 75, 86
bites 17, 34, 38, 60, 81–2
black pepper 91
blood pressure, 23, 76–7
'Blue Grass' (perfume) 9
boils 47–8
borage oil 42
broad-leaved lavender 111
bronchitis 38, 80, 113
bruises 17, 54–5
bumps 54–5
burns 17, 18, 19, 34, 55–6

camphor 112, 113
carbuncles 56
carrier oils 41, 42
Cassidony stoechas 113
chamomile 52, 54, 60, 64, 69, 70,

73, 81, 83, 91, 92, 93,
99, 100, 104
chamomile roman 107
chest complaints 10
chickenpox 56–8
childbirth 95–7
children xiii, 43–4, 58–60
cicitrizant properties 17, 33–4, 102
cineole 112
cinnamon leaf 97
circulation problems 36
citronella 82
civilisation diseases 104–5
clary sage 93, 99
clove 97
cold sores 74
colds 80
colic 58, 59, 112
compresses 39–40
concretes 113
constituents 30–32, 115–17
convulsions 14
cosmetic preparations 34, 102–3
cradle cap 60
cramp 14, 34, 37, 90
Culpeper, Nicholas 13–14
cuts 34, 58, 60, 61–2
cypress 52
cystitis 38, 63–4

decontractant agent 34
deodorant properties 34, 94
depression xvi, 16, 35–6, 64–5
dermatitis 65–7
detergents 30
diaper rash 59
diaphoretic effects 38
digestive problems 11, 14, 36
dihydrolinalool 32
Dioscorides 3, 10
disinfectant uses 7, 18, 43, 67–8
distillation 4–6, 28–9
douches 42
dropsy 14
dyspepsia *see* indigestion

earache 34, 69
eczema 34, 65–7
electric diffusers 43
Elizabeth I, Queen 13
emmenagogic properties 18
emotional stress 37
epilepsy 70, 112
essential oil:
  history 4–6
  production 27–32
esters 30, 31, 112
eucalyptus 68, 81, 82, 85
evening primrose oil 98
expectorant properties 112

fainting 14
falling sickness 13, 14
fatigue 70–71
feet, bathing 39
fenchone 113
fennel 52, 97
fever 38
flatulence 68–9, 112
fleas 42, 81, 94–5
flu 80
frankincense 54
French lavender 10, 11, 113
frostbite 61
fungicidal qualities 38
furuncle 47–8

Galen 10
gangrene 19
gargling 40
garlic 64, 80
Gattefossé René Maurice 18–19
genital herpes 74–5
genito-urinary infections 38, 42
geranium 54, 99, 103
Gerard, John 13
germicidal properties 16
ginger 52
gout 51–2
grapeseed oil 41
Grieve, M. 16
gum infections 40

haemorrhoids 96
hair care 42, 71–3
hands, bathing 39
harmonizing properties 35
hazelnut oil 42
Heacham, Norfolk 29
headaches 16, 73–4, 112
healing, historical use 10–15
heart rate 24
herbal medicine xiv–xv, 10–15,
        16, 43
herpes 74–5
Hildegarde, Abbess 11–12
horsefly bites 81
hospitals, use in 21–5
hyperactivity 35, 59
hypertension 35, 76–7
hyssop 97
hysteria 35, 89
immune system 36, 77–9, 104
immuno-stimulant properties 38
impetigo 79
indigestion 34, 37, 68–9
infectious illnesses 79–81, 112
inhalation 20, 40
insect bites *see* bites
insect repellent 38, 43, 81
insecticide properties 38
insomnia 20, 21, 22–3, 59, 82–3
internal use, not advised 44

jasmine 65
jetlag 83–4
jojoba oil 41
juniper 52, 97

ketones 112, 113

Labiatae xii, 17, 26
labour pain 96–7
laryngitis 84–5
lavandin xvi, 24, 111, 112–13,
        114
*Lavandula angustifolia* xii, xiv, 24,
        26, 112, 113
*L. a.* 'Aroma' 114
*L. a.* 'Bowles Early' 114

*L. a.* 'Dwarf Blue' 114
*L. a.* 'Hemus' 113
*L. a.* 'Hidcote Pink' 114
*L. a.* 'Karlovo' 113
*L. a.* 'Kazanluc' 113
*L. a.* Mill. 111
*L. a.* 'Svezhest' 114
*L. burnatii* 24, 112
*L. delphinensis* 113
*L. fragrans* 113
*L. hortensis* 112
*L. hybrida* 112
*L. latifolia* xvi, 111, 112
*L. officinalis* xii, xvi, 26
*L. o.* Chaix 26
*L. spica* 111
*L. stoechas* 10, 11, 111, 113
*L. vera* xii, xvi, 11
*L. v.* de Canolle 26
*L. x intermedia* xvi, 111, 112
lavender 'abrial' 112–13
lavender 'reydovan' 112
lavender water 6, 8, 30, 34, 42,
        93–4
'Lavender' (Yardley perfume) 9
lemon 52, 68
lemongrass 82
lesser lavender 111
leucorrhoea 85–6
lice 12, 42, 86–7, 95
linalool 30–31, 32, 112
linalyl acetate 31

marjoram 52, 81, 90, 93, 97, 100
masks 42
massage xv, 20, 41, 58–9, 76–7
Maury, Marguerite 19–20
melissa 67
Mencière, Dr 17
menopause 87–8
menstrual problems 11, 14
Merton Priory 27
migraine 13, 88
Mitcham, Surrey 27–9
moisturizers 102–3
mood swings 89

mosquito bites 81
mosquito repellent 38
moth repellent 4, 5, 38, 81
mouth infections 40
mucolytic properties 112
muscle tension 21
muscular aches and pains xiii, 34, 89–91
muscular spasms 21, 34, 37, 90
myrrh 61, 97

naga sores 108–9
nappy rash 59
*Nardus italica* 111
National Lavender Collection 114
nausea 91
neat application 40
neroli 51, 65, 67, 92, 99
nerve tonic 20
nervous problems 13
nervous system, regulating effect 35–7

Old English Lavender xvi

'Paco Rabanne' (perfume) 9
pain relief 20–21, 23, 34, 96–7
palpitations 35, 91–2
parasiticidal properties 38
parasympathetic nervous system 37
Parkinson, John 13
patchouli 61
peach oil 42
pediculosis 86–7
peppermint 91, 97, 101
perfumes 7–9, 34, 93–4, 113
period pains 34, 92–3
perspiration, excessive 94
pesticide properties 18
pet care 94–5
pillows, herbal xiii, 4, 5, 82
pine 52
Pliny the Elder 10–11
postnatal depression 97
pot-pourri xiii, 4, 5
poultices 39–40
pregnancy, use 43–4, 95–7

premenstrual tension 97–9
preventative properties 38
production 26–32
prophylactic properties 38
pruritis 85–6
psoriasis 61
psychosomatic disease 36

rashes 95
regulating effects 35–7
rejuvenating properties 19–20, 34
relaxation 95
respiration 25
respiratory infections xvi, 38, 40, 113
restlessness 37, 59
restorative properties 35
rheumatism 34, 99–100, 112
rose 51, 54, 65, 92, 99, 103
rosemary 17, 52, 73, 84, 91, 97, 100
Rovesti, Prof. Paolo 35–6

safety 43–4
sage 17, 97
Salmon, William 14
sandalwood 64, 86
scabies 100–101
scalds 17
scarring, prevention 18, 62, 102
scratches 61–2
sedative effects 18, 20–24, 36, 50, 112
shingles 57
shock 101–2
'Silvestre' (perfume) 9
sinusitis 113
sitz baths 42
skin:
  blemishes 60
  care 20, 33–4, 42, 102–3
  cleanser 102
  complaints xvi
  cracked 61
  strengthener for acid mantle 103
  toner 102
sleeping difficulties *see* insomnia

snake bites 11
soap 8, 30, 113
soothing remedy 34
sore throats 80
sores 17, 58, 62
soya oil 41
spasms 21, 34, 37, 90
spike lavender xvi, 14, 27,
      111–13, 114
splinters, infected 103–4
spots 34, 48–9, 60
sprains 104
steam distillation 29
steam inhalation 40
stichados 113
stickadore 113
stimulating properties 112
stings 34, 38, 58, 81–2
stoechas lavender 111
storage 44
stress-related conditions 20, 24,
      35–7, 104–7
stretch marks 96
sunburn 107
sunflower oil 41
sweet almond oil 41
sweet waters 5, 6
sympathetic nervous system 37

tachycardia 91–2
tea tree 32, 48, 49, 52, 55, 56,
      58, 61, 62, 64, 67, 68,
      73, 77, 78, 82, 85, 86,
      87, 90, 94, 95, 100, 101,
      103, 104, 107, 109
teas xiii, 5
teething 59–60
terracotta oil burners 43
therapeutic effects 24–5
thyme 17, 97

tonic effects xiii, 36
toothache 14, 34
travel sickness 91
tropical ulcers 108–9
true lavender xii, xvi, 11, 111,
      112–13, 114
tummy ache 58, 59
Turner, William 13
types 24, 32, 111–14

ulcers 108–9
urethritis 63–4
uterine disorders 10

vaginal infections 42, 85–6
valerian 83
Valnet, Dr Jean 17–18
vaporization 43, 58–9
varicose ulcers 17, 19, 108–9
venereal sores 19
vermifuge properties 38
vertigo 101–2
Victoria, Queen 6
vinegar 5
vitamin B6 98
vitamin B complex 98
vitamin C 80
voice, loss of 14

wasp stings 81
water distillation 28–9
West Indian bay 73
wheatgerm oil 41
whooping cough 109
wound-healing properties 16–17,
      19, 33–4, 61–2, 102
wounds 61–2

Yardley 8–9, 29–30
ylang ylang 51, 70, 92

zona 57